*Communication
between doctors
and patients*

Communication between doctors and patients

Contributors: Colin Fraser, Marie Johnston, Peter Maguire, Derek Rutter, Philip Ley, and Martin Fishbein

EDITED BY A. E. BENNETT

Published for the
Nuffield Provincial Hospitals Trust
by the Oxford University Press

Published for the Nuffield Provincial Hospitals Trust
3 Prince Albert Road, London NW1 7SP
by Oxford University Press

Oxford London Glasgow New York
Toronto Melbourne Wellington Cape Town
Ibadan Nairobi Dar es Salaam Lusaka Addis Ababa
Kuala Lumpur Singapore Jakarta Hong Kong Tokyo
Delhi Bombay Calcutta Madras Karachi

ISBN 0 19 721392 8

© The Nuffield Provincial Hospitals Trust 1976

Designed by Bernard Crossland
Printed in Great Britain
by Hazell Watson & Viney Limited
Aylesbury, Bucks

Contents

Foreword

The invitation which I received from the Trustees of the Nuffield Provincial Hospitals Trust in 1971 to write a monograph on *Communication in Medicine* led me to study in far greater detail than I would ever have done otherwise the art and science of a technique at which I, and I am sure most of my professional colleagues, were confident that they were proficient. My study led me to realize not only how ill-founded this confidence was, but also how necessary it is for the efficient and kindly practice of medicine that doctors should learn how to communicate with their patients, their colleagues, and the public better than most of them manage to do today.

One of the suggestions I made to promote recognition of this need was that steps should be taken to provide a forum to encourage improved methods of communication which might possibly take the form of an association for the study of communication in medicine. This suggestion received a cautious welcome from the Secretary of the Trust and he rightly considered that before any formal attempt was made to launch such an association it would be desirable that the idea should be discussed in greater detail by a group of interested people, both medically qualified and lay.

A meeting with this purpose was held in October 1973 and the group concluded that it would be useful to discover what sort of worthwhile recent developments there had been in this area and what studies were being undertaken. For if there was little work in progress there would be little to report to and discuss at meetings of any larger association of interested people. Dr A. E. Bennett was asked to undertake these explorations and in December 1974 a slightly enlarged group assembled to hear a presentation of some of the work which he had discovered and considered most relevant to the basic problems of interpersonal communication in medicine. The group found the investigations which were then reported so interesting and stimulating that they proposed that more detailed reports of the work that had been informally presented to them should be prepared for publication by the Trust. It was also suggested that when the book was ready for publication its contents should be presented for discussion to a wider invited audience which should also be asked to consider the idea that some permanent group or association should be formed to stimulate the prosecution and regular presentation and debate of further studies of this and related kinds.

And here, in this volume, are the papers which excited the enthusiastic interest of the informal group to whom they were first presented. They give a glimpse into great and largely untapped opportunities for research and study, not only into the fundamental skills which are needed to facilitate communication between individuals but also into the important benefits which improved communication could contribute to both teaching and practice of good clinical and administrative medicines.

I do not think it is fanciful to forecast that if this initiative of the Nuffield Provincial Hospitals Trust were vigorously pursued, doctors and their colleagues in future generations might look back at our present primitive understanding of how to communicate with each other and with our patients and the public about medical matters with as much pity and incredulity as we now look back at the therapeutic poverty of our predecessors. This forecast, of course, could only be fulfilled if the need for improved communications became more widely recognized and if the manifold opportunities for basic and applied research were to attract the vigorous interest of original thinkers in every branch of our National Health Service.

C.M.FLETCHER
CBE, MD, FRCP, FFCM

Royal Postgraduate Medical School
London W12
December 1975

Acknowledgements

I should like to express, on behalf of all contributors, thanks to Professor Charles Fletcher for acting as our chairman and providing the stimulus responsible for both the seminar and this book; Mr Gordon McLachlan and Mr Dick Shegog for their interest and encouragement and providing the opportunity for presenting and discussing our work; those who attended the seminar and challenged us by their discussion; and lastly our secretaries who have borne the brunt of our labours.

We are indebted to the Nuffield Provincial Hospitals Trust for their support.

A.E.BENNETT

Contributors

A. E. Bennett, MB, FFCM. Professor of Clinical Epidemiology and Social Medicine, St George's Hospital Medical School, London SW17.

C. Fraser, MA, PHD. University Lecturer in Social Psychology, Social and Political Sciences Committee, University of Cambridge.

M. Fishbein, BA, PHD. Professor of Psychology and Research Professor, Institute of Communications Research, University of Illinois, Urbana-Champaign.

M. Johnston, BSC, PHD. Research Officer, Health Services Evaluation Group, Department of the Regius Professor of Medicine, University of Oxford.

P. Ley, BA, PHD. Senior Lecturer in Clinical Psychology, Sub-department of Clinical Psychology, Department of Psychiatry, University of Liverpool.

P. Maguire, BA, MB, MRCPSYCH, DPM. Senior Lecturer, Department of Psychiatry, University of Manchester: formerly Clinical Tutor in Psychiatry, University of Oxford.

D. Rutter, BA, PHD. Research Psychologist, Department of Psychiatry, University of Oxford.

Preamble

The papers which follow are based on those presented to an invited audience at a one-day seminar arranged by the Nuffield Provincial Hospitals Trust as part of a follow-up to Professor Charles Fletcher's Rock Carling Monograph, *Communication in Medicine*.[1] Those present were drawn from many disciplines and represented a diversity of interests. Since I helped in the planning of the programme, I must try to describe the purpose of the seminar and now of this book. But first I feel I should describe how I came to be involved.

My entry into the subject of communications in medicine came about from a narrow interest in the design and use of questionnaires in research and clinical settings. In preparing a monograph on this subject,[2] I helped write the following introductory paragraphs:

> The aim of the questionnaire designer is to communicate with potential respondents using the medium of the questionnaire. It is his responsibility to ensure that questions can be fully understood and that the respondent is encouraged to reciprocate in this communication process. For this it is important that the researcher understand something of the nature of this communication process, and thus appreciate the task that he is setting the respondent.
>
> Responding is not a simple stimulus-response process but a complex procedure by which the respondent selects a small amount of his total information to become the questionnaire data. Each question will alert the respondent in a particular direction, causing him to focus on some aspect of his total experience. The relevant experience may be well thought out and organized in his mind, though more likely it will be vague and

1. Fletcher, C. M., *Communication in Medicine*, Rock Carling Monograph (London: Nuffield Provincial Hospitals Trust, 1973).
2. Bennett, A. E., and Ritchie, K., *Questionnaires in Medicine: A Guide to their Design and Use* (Oxford University Press for the Nuffield Provincial Hospitals Trust, 1975).

confused due to the limitation of memory. The effect of memory may well vary according to the nature of the information. Unfortunately however, the process of forgetting cannot be predicted for memory is selective and the process by which information is stored or discarded is influenced by incidental emotional factors as well as the continual process of extinction. Furthermore, memory is seldom an all-or-none event. Experience may be remembered in a distorted or incomplete form, confusing events and magnifying them out of their original proportions. Additionally the relevant experience may have become associated in time with other experiences so that the question brings to mind a much broader range of ideas than is relevant.

This complex of ideas must then be brought into full awareness—a process complicated by such psychological phenomena as self-analysis, conceptualization of ideas, and generalization from specific points. The respondent is thus forming a percept of his own ideas and the process of producing this percept may be affected by wishful thinking, a desire to please the research worker and the desire to be fair to oneself and to others, and will probably be accompanied by a good deal of confusion. The respondent then has to decide what aspects of all this information he is prepared to communicate. He may be reluctant to communicate information which is embarrassing or socially unacceptable. He may have misgivings as to the purpose for which his information will be used and the conclusions that might be drawn from it. Working against this censoring procedure will be forces motivating the respondent to answer fully and thoughtfully. This positive motivation derives from two sources. First, a desire to influence his present state, where the questioner is seen as someone able to bring about changes for the respondent's benefit. Secondly, there is the gratification which the respondent receives from the communication process itself.

Perhaps only then did I fully appreciate the enormity of the subject and my own ignorance. It led me to the notion that in general those who know anything about communication in a theoretical sense are not closely involved in trying to improve it in everyday medical situations: conversely those of us interested in improving this aspect of our work most often do not have the necessary theoretical knowledge. The reasons for this are not difficult to find.

Recent years have seen the volume of scientific research into human communication escalating rapidly. This activity is due to ever-increasing interest in and use of the term communication and to numerous scientific disciplines staking their claims. The physical sciences contribute by way of cybernetics, information theory, and general systems theory. The social sciences identify, for example, the interests of anthropologists, sociologists, experimental and social psychologists, and may be extended to include the interests of linguists who describe their work on language structure as part of communication science. Out of all this activity has come more than twenty different concepts of the word communication but there is yet to be established an acceptable definition. The field has been described as a teeming wilderness of facts and notions, instances and generalizations, proofs and surmises, and a jungle of unrelated concepts and a mass of undigested, often sterile, empirical data.

However, some sort of definition is necessary. For our purposes I think the term communication is best defined as a 'process by which senders and receivers of messages interact in given social contexts'. Thus no single aspect of communication can be meaningfully understood when parted from the other constituents of behaviour. Further, as the responses of the communicators are included, the notion of interaction cannot be considered as a one-way transmission process.

With this background I should now like to comment on our plan and purpose. The papers are designed in an attempt to produce a framework for the consideration of interpersonal communication in the most common situation of medicine, face-to-face contact between doctor, therapist, or nurse, and patient. To aid discussion of this framework, there are examples from past and current work, starting narrowly and broadening. Then, to avoid any false sense of security, the dimensions of attitude and behaviour change are added.

This is the plan which by its very nature must draw extensively on disciplines other than medicine. The purpose is more difficult to describe. Charles Fletcher in his Rock Carling Monograph on *Communication in Medicine*[1] described a somewhat unhappy state of affairs. This raised the questions of whether things are as bad as described, and more importantly, what should be done. For simply describing a bad situation does not necessarily identify what we should do. To this end in his monograph he laid down certain

1. Fletcher, C. M., *Communication in Medicine*. Rock Carling Monograph (London: Nuffield Provincial Hospitals Trust, 1973).

principles of communication and I should like to repeat these here. They are:

1. The purpose of communication is not just to deliver a message but to effect a change in the recipient in respect of his knowledge, his attitude, or eventually, in his behaviour.

2. The value of a communication is to be judged not on its purpose or content but on its effect on the recipient. An elegant or witty communication may satisfy the communicator but leave the recipient uninformed and unmoved.

3. Good communication is difficult. Few can master it without special tuition and constant attention to its effectiveness.

4. Communication must be matched to the knowledge, social background, interest, purposes, and needs of the recipient. It requires empathy, which is 'the power of projecting one's personality into, and so fully understanding, the object of contemplation'.

5. Communication is effected not only by words, which must have the same meaning for giver and receiver, but also by attitudes, expressions, and gestures. This is especially relevant to a consultation where patient and doctor are both givers and receivers.

6. If communication is to change behaviour, the required change in the recipient must be seen by him to have more advantages than drawbacks; otherwise it will not be made, or if it is made, will not persist. New information resulting in a change of attitude is usually a necessary prelude to a change in behaviour.

7. To make sure that a communication has succeeded, information about its effects ('feedback') both immediate or subsequent is needed.

8. Communication demands effort, thought, time, and often money. Effective communication between colleagues also demands willingness on the part of the giver to discover that more may be learnt than taught.

Unfortunately he did not, and in all fairness could not, within the scope and length of his book, develop these further. As a result much remained unsaid. What follows is really an exploration of these principles; an attempt to see how much more we need to know in order to be able to tackle the problems before us in an informed and concerted manner.

A.E. BENNETT

An analysis of face-to-face communication

Colin Fraser
Lecturer in Social Psychology
University of Cambridge

An analysis of
face-to-face communication

I should like to present an analysis of face-to-face communication in terms of four *systems* which are used for three distinguishable *types* of communication, and then discuss briefly the question of communication effectiveness. But first an introductory comment.

As a social psychologist, I am aware of two quite different traditions or frameworks for the study of interpersonal communication. The older tradition, reviewed in detail by William McGuire (1968), developed in connection with work on attitude and behaviour change. Typically, an investigator would measure an attitude or behaviour, then produce a persuasive communication in an attempt to induce change, and then assess the attitude and behaviour once more. Work in this tradition has told us about many of the precursors and consequences of communications, but let me suggest that one of its major weaknesses has been that it has never told us a great deal about the nature of the communications themselves. The second, much more recent, one might be called the socio-linguistic approach, and this has started to analyse the communication *per se* in great detail, but as yet has relatively little to say about other, broader issues. My paper is clearly within, and limited to, this second framework.

Let me introduce my analysis with a developmental example. If a friend told you, 'You're an idiot', but said this with a smile, you might well feel the assertion was not intended to be as unfriendly as it seems in print. In fact, you might treat it as a joke, in which the positive and negative elements just about cancel each other out. But such a combination coming from a *woman* would be interpreted by a child as distinctly negative and unfriendly, according to Bugental and her colleagues (1970), who carried out an intricate study in which they used a number of messages each composed of three separable components: (*a*) a verbal component, for example, 'You really did a fine job'; (*b*) a vocal or 'intonational' component; (*c*) a visual or facial component. They were then able to produce messages consisting of all possible combinations of positive and negative (friendly and unfriendly) verbal, vocal, and visual components. Their study raises a number of points of interest for us.

It immediately reminds us that language, the most familiar and most studied of the human systems of communication is not the only form of communication operating in face-to-face interaction. In fact, when we use language we normally use it accompanied by, or embedded in, a rich multi-system context, and it would be surprising if the different systems did not interact in the encoding and decoding of communications. Bugental's study raises a number of questions about the detailed description of face-to-face communication. How many systems of communication are there? How are they organized? How do different systems interact? Such questions will be discussed in the section on four systems of communication, where the emphasis will be on 'communication as behaviour'. There we shall be particularly concerned with describing the observable behaviour or the overt forms of the messages that occur during communication. But Bugental's study also implies other questions. Do different systems serve the same or different functions? What information is transmitted by the systems? What is the meaning of the communicative behaviours? These questions focus on 'communication as meaning', which will be the emphasis of the section on three types of communication.

Study of the overt form, or surface structure, of communication is necessary but not sufficient in itself for explaining the meanings or understandings that are communicated, as can be illustrated from Bugental's work. She found that the exact meaning of a combination of components varied with the nature of the participants involved in the message encoding or decoding. Thus, the same set of components could mean different things depending on whether an adult or a child decoded the message, and in addition the meaning of the set of components differed for the child depending on whether a man or a woman produced the message. (For the children, a smile from a man 'cancelled out' accompanying negative verbal and vocal components, but a female smile failed to do so.)

Thus, communication involves relating the overt forms of messages to the participants in the encounter. But it entails much more than this. Hymes (1972) has claimed that we must take into account at least sixteen different 'components of speech' if we are to understand how spoken language is used in communication. These components, which include features of message forms, aspects of social settings, and mixtures of the two, can be collapsed into eight major categories which, Hymes ingeniously proposes, can be remembered by the mnemonic SPEAKING. Thus, 'S' stands for 'setting', or 'scene', which includes times, place, and physical characteristics of the situation, as well as the 'psychological setting' or cultural definition of the occasion. 'P' stands for 'participants', who may be speakers, intended addressees, hearers, members of an audience, and the like. 'E' refers to 'ends', or purposes of interactions, such as whether the aim is to issue an invitation, engage in an argument, or accomplish a co-operative task. In combination, these three major categories largely account for what is often termed the social setting, or context, of messages, and the interrelations of behaviour and the settings in which it occurs gets us much nearer an understanding of meanings. But as will become clear by the end of this paper, perhaps there is even more to communication than that. First, however, let us turn to the task of describing the observables of communication.

Four communication systems

In this section I shall introduce a number of basic concepts in the study of linguistic and non-linguistic communication and, it is hoped, reveal the richness of the behaviour involved in conversation, the prime exemplar of human communication.

I shall focus on behaviours which are parts of socially shared signal systems or codes, the use of which entails intentional encoding and decoding. This ignores many isolated actions, idiosyncratic acts, and signals which might be given an interpretation by an observer but could hardly be said to have been encoded; if every tic, pimple, and egg-stained tie becomes a 'communication', then 'communication' itself becomes an all-encompassing, uninformative term. The descriptions of the different systems that contribute to a conversation will necessarily be brief. Fuller accounts of the structure of language are available in an introductory text in linguistics (for example, Langacre, 1968; Crystal, 1971); more detailed descriptions of the non-linguistic systems can be found in Argyle (1969) and Laver and Hutcheson (1972). Note that I suggest it is convenient to analyse language into two major components, the verbal and the intonational, and for simplicity of exposition I shall describe each as a system in its own right.

The verbal system

Obviously speech depends on sounds and it is probably the case that no two sounds produced by a speaker are ever completely identical. Normally, however, we ignore many variations in duration, aspiration, and the like and treat all b sounds, for example, as if they were the same. All languages appear to operate with a limited number, usually several dozen, of such basic classes of sounds, or phonemes, which are not meaningful in themselves, but are lawfully combined into longer segments and then meaning enters the picture. The smallest meaningful unit in a language is a 'morpheme' which can be a short word, or part of a word; all words contain at least one morpheme, but all morphemes are not complete words. For example, 'chair' is one morpheme because it cannot be broken into smaller meaningful units, but 'chairman' consists of two morphemes, and 'chairmanship' consists of three.

With the units of 'morpheme' and 'word' we enter the domain of grammar and semantics. Grammar describes the structuring of morphemes into words and words into longer sequences, whereas semantics organizes the content of morphemes and words and relates them to the non-linguistic world about which the verbal system is being used to communicate. A semantic analysis of language tells us much, but not everything, about the meaning of what is said, because as we have seen, meaning is also derived from the social setting, and, as we shall see, from implicit, difficult to pin down, shared understandings and common backgrounds. Lawfully, morphemes are combined into words, words into larger phrases and clauses, and these, in turn, into units we shall call 'utterances'. An utterance can be thought of as a sentence-like chunk, which is used to express something approximating one whole idea. Notice, however, that many common types of utterances in conversation do not correspond to conventional notions of a sentence standing in isolation. Depending on what has been said before or on what is self-evident in the situation, sentence fragments can be acceptable utterances. For example, in response to the appropriate question, virtually any word, phrase, or clause could constitute an entire utterance.

In the past, it has often been implied that the largest structural unit of language is the single sentence, or utterance, and it is only recently that linguists have felt themselves in a position to start doing justice to the regularities that extend beyond the boundaries of single utterances (for example, Sinclair and Coulthard, 1975). The analysis of such regularities is called 'discourse analysis' and the structural dependencies from utterance to utterance are often termed 'cohesion'. One common form of cohesion, for example, is the use of pronouns, and another is sequence signals, such as 'thus', 'therefore', 'nevertheless'. One further, and particularly important, cohesive device is ellipsis. If someone asks me, 'Do you have change for a parking meter?', I am more likely to follow rules of ellipsis and reply, 'Yes, I have', or 'Yes, I think so', than to respond with the full-blown sentence, 'Yes, I do have change for a parking meter'. Making use of such structural features of everyday speech, Sinclair and Coulthard (1975) have proposed that the utterances of the classroom, and probably of many other settings, too, can be organized in terms of a hierarchy of successive higher-order units. The development of such discourse analyses will prove very helpful for the understanding of conversation and communication, particularly if they can indicate cohesion, or lack of cohesion, across the contributions of different speakers.

Intonation

What has been described so far is not, even schematically, a complete description of spoken language. Rather, it corresponds approximately to those features of speech which are conventionally preserved in written form, primarily the words. But, in speaking, this verbal system is completely combined with, or overlaid by, the systematic use of different pitches, stresses, and junctures. It is not the words themselves which tell us whether, 'You think they'll be all right', is to be taken as a declarative or an interrogative, but a drop or rise in pitch at the end of the utterance. Similarly, it is not the words which distinguish a 'black board' from a 'blackboard' or 'lighthousekeeping' from 'light housekeeping'. The distinctions are dependent primarily on differences in stress patterns.

The intonational system is composed of patterns of pitch and stress, with junctures marking the boundaries of the units over which pitch and stress are interacting. Systematic changes in intonation mark systematic changes in meaning within utterances. Intonation also affects larger units of discourse. For example, quite a subtle form of cohesion across utterances is the use of emphasis. If you joined a conversation just in time to hear someone say, 'John's car is *blue*', with a marked stress on 'blue', you could assume that previously someone had claimed it was some other colour.

The study of intonation has not been as well developed as that of the verbal system, but it is clear that the two interact very closely, and together they comprise spoken language. To complicate matters, however, there is a further vocal system, which is not generally regarded as linguistic, that is as forming part of language *per se*.

Paralinguistics

When we vocalize we do more than use the verbal and intonational systems of language (see Birdwhistell, 1961: Abercrombie, 1968). We also produce a variety of additional vocalizations, some of which, at least, are culturally determined, shared by members of a given social group and used communicatively. These include 'ums' and 'ahs', coughs, splutters, giggles, and the like. Other paralinguistic phenomena are usually held to be responsible for the ill-defined notion of 'tone of voice'. They include extremes of intensity, pitch and drawl, including yelling and whispering. Laughing and crying, moaning and groaning, whining, yawning, and even belching are also paralinguistic elements.

In addition, paralinguistics can be thought to cover phenomena relating to the timing of speech, and to the use of silence in speech, particularly in the form of pauses or hesitation phenomena. A distinction usually drawn here is between unfilled (or silent) pauses and filled pauses, involving sounds like 'um', 'ah', and 'er'. Various functions have been proposed for hesitation phenomena. They may be used by the speaker to discourage interruptions and to keep the floor. They may permit and indicate planning of speech. Or they may be indices of anxiety. Precisely which phenomena fulfil which functions is still open to dispute (Cook, 1971). Some features of hesitation, timing, and speech rate may well be primarily idiosyncratic elements of personal style. Like stable features of voice quality, these can provide what Laver (1968) has called indexical information, that is information about supposed characteristics of the speaker, without being part of a shared system for communication.

Kinesics

This term will be used to describe body and facial movements, many of which have now been shown to occur in culturally standardized forms with clear communicative significance. One investigator

(Sheflen, 1964) has argued, for example, that there are only about thirty traditional American gestures and an even smaller number of postural configurations of communicative importance for Americans. The same investigator has claimed that, at least in psychiatric interviews, posture and body movement is used to mark different phases or units of the interaction. Between the relatively small unit of a single verbal utterance and the complete interaction, which he termed a 'presentation', Sheflen identified two intermediate-sized units. Several utterances formed a 'point' whose beginning and end were marked by shifts in head posture. Several successive points constituted a 'position', or phase lasting up to five or six minutes. Beginnings and ends of 'positions' were indicated by gross shifts in posture, such as changing from sitting forward to leaning back in a chair. It would be interesting to know if such kinesic changes are emphasizing features in the interaction which discourse analysis could show are also being conveyed linguistically.

Such seems to be a primary function of hand movements (Argyle, 1969). Although hand movements, in large part, are socially shared and vary from society to society (Efron, 1941), it has proved difficult as yet to provide a useful set of categories to describe the variety and richness of them. Like hand movements, head movements are highly visible, but unlike the former, their variations are limited. Nevertheless, head nods and shakes can convey important information about the listener's attentiveness, agreement, and encouragement for the speaker to continue. The fact that in certain societies nods and shakes mean the reverse of what they mean in English-speaking countries (Leach, 1972) indicates that head movements constitute a learned, socially shared, though simple, system of communication.

Facial movements can be analysed in great detail. According to Vine (1969) one form of traditional Indian theatre makes use of six standard eyebrow positions and twenty-eight eye positions. A more recent analysis of naturalistic behaviour (Birdwhistell, 1968) described four eyebrow positions, four eyelid positions, and seven positions of the mouth. Presumably, it is to configurations of such minute facial movements that people react when they infer emotions from facial expressions.

One particularly interesting set of head and facial movements are those involved in gazing at another person and in mutal eye-contact (Argyle and Cook, 1975). They can help communicate one type of relationship rather than another, such as an asexual friendship or a much more sexually oriented one. In addition, gaze and eye-contact play an important part in regulating conversation and will be discussed in more detail as part of 'interaction regulation'. Indeed, it can be argued (Argyle, 1969) that the face is second only to the voice in what is called, after all, face-to-face communication.

During a conversation, the kinesic, paralinguistic, and linguistic elements are constantly changing and hence can be described as 'dynamic features' of the interaction. They are changing, however, against a more constant background to the conversation, made up of what Argyle and Kendon (1967) have termed 'standing features'. These relatively unchanging aspects of an interaction, such as proximity and appearance of the participants, can themselves be used to communicate. The distance or seating arrangements between two people can be a clear, and shared, index of the relationship between them or of the type of communication, public or private, for example, that they are currently engaged in. Much the same can be said of the dress and grooming of the participants. For completeness sake, it is useful to bear in mind these standing features.

Relations between systems

An analysis of face-to-face communication in terms of the four different systems is a first step in revealing the richness and intricacy of human communication processes. It is also a useful basis for understanding several simpler analyses, which though sometimes used interchangeably, are in fact confusingly different. By now, it should be clear that when communication is divided into the verbal and non-verbal, as social psychologists tend to do, this is not the same as splitting it into linguistic and non-linguistic components. Furthermore, neither of those distinctions corresponds to an analysis in terms of the two major channels of communication, defined by the sensory-motor apparatus involved. Table 1 illustrates these differing distinctions, and reveals that whereas all three of them agree in separating the verbal from the kinesic, they apportion the intonational and the paralinguistic quite differently.

Normally the different systems operate in a compatible and supportive fashion. A person arguing that something is particularly important, is likely to use both verbal and intonational means to do so, and it is unlikely that paralinguistic or kinesic cues would indicate boredom or flippancy. It is improbable that a conveyor of sad news

Table 1. *Varying classifications of the four communication systems*

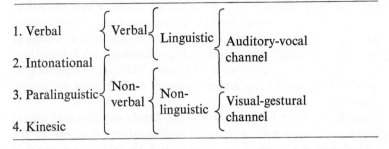

1. Verbal	Verbal	Linguistic	Auditory-vocal channel
2. Intonational			
3. Paralinguistic	Non-verbal	Non-linguistic	Visual-gestural channel
4. Kinesic			

will sound or look happy. The non-linguistic systems, particularly head and hand-movements, are often used to support, emphasize, or 'punctuate' the linguistic elements. One might in fact be tempted to assume that compared to the linguistic systems, the non-linguistic ones are relatively unimportant, and such a view would appear to receive strong support from Moscovici (1967). After discussing a study he had conducted in which he had detected no differences between ordinary face-to-face conversations and face-to-face conversations with an opaque screen between the participants, Moscovici concluded that in the screen situation, 'the suppression of non-linguistic signals had no marked effect; participants conversed as though gestures, body movement, and facial expressions did not normally play a major role in communication or serve as cues for transmitting information.'

But before concluding that language invariably dominates face-to-face communication it is as well to consider what happens when the systems do not appear to be in agreement. Bugental's study is one instance. Others have been conducted by Argyle and his colleagues. Argyle *et al.* (1970) studied the relative effects of verbal and non-verbal variations conveying superiority, neutrality, or inferiority of the speaker. They concluded that the non-verbal cues, which involved 'tones of voice', facial expressions, and head-orientations, were much more important than the verbal ones. At best, with compatible components, the verbal components strengthened the perceived nature of the message. When the components were in conflict, the verbal cues were more or less ineffective. Over-all, they estimated that the non-verbal cues had several times the effect of the verbal cues on subjects' responses.

The resolution of this apparent contradiction concerning the importance of linguistic and non-linguistic systems is not hard to find, and has been hinted at at various points above. When Moscovici claimed that various non-linguistic components had little role to play in communication or in transmitting information, in the context in which he wrote the 'information' being transmitted was information about the topic of discussion, namely films. This type of communication can be thought of as 'representational' or 'ideational' or 'propositional' communication.

But this was not being assessed in the Argyle and Bugental studies which were concerned with the communication to others of the attitudes of the speakers, with what can be called 'interpersonal communication'. Particularly when systems were in conflict, they found the non-verbal (perhaps especially the non-linguistic) systems conveyed most information about the superior/inferior, friendly/hostile attitudes of the speaker. But they were not concerned with what was being discussed while those attitudes prevailed; that the linguistic systems made clear. It is possible that non-linguistic cues alone could not distinguish between superiority (or friendliness) manifested in the context of a discussion about the existence of God, the conduct of a clinical interview, or the price of sausages.

So communication systems can be used to communicate about the topic or about the attitudes and relations of the participants. A related distinction has, in the past, been conveyed by contrasting language as 'message' and as 'expressive behaviour'. But a third focus of communication can occur, the conversation itself. Irrespective of what is being discussed or the attitudes of the participants, the speakers are likely to communicate in order to maintain and control the conversation. This third type of communication can be called 'interaction regulation'.

Halliday (1973) has drawn related distinctions amongst three 'language functions'; the ideational, the interpersonal, and the textual. The fact that Halliday's discussions were centred on language alone conveniently reminds us that language can be used not just for representational information but for all three types of communication. Think of, 'You're a louse' and 'Let me finish, then you can have your say'. Similarly, non-linguistic systems can convey representational information, as well as play major roles in interpersonal communication and interaction regulation. A combination of gestures, head, and eye movements could make quite clear, for example, who is to move which piece of furniture into which room. So, to some extent, different communication systems can substitute for one another, and can be used for each of the three types of communication.

Nevertheless there do seem to be clear differences in emphasis regarding what type of communication is normally carried out by the different systems. Representational communication is largely the province of language, with its systematic grammatical structure and intricate semantic mapping on to the non-linguistic world. On the other hand, a great deal of interaction regulation is non-linguistic. All systems can readily be demonstrated to convey interpersonal information, although particularly when systems appear to be in conflict about interpersonal meanings—about, for example, what people's attitudes towards each other are—then we seem to pay more attention to paralinguistic and kinesic cues than to what is overtly being said. It is as if information, often allowed to remain submerged because it is not too important, is seen in these situations to leak out and float to the surface (Ekman and Friesen, 1969).

Three types of communication

In this section, I shall use some important studies to provide brief illustrations of each of the three types of communication.

Interaction regulation

The form a conversation takes is determined, in part, before the conversation itself begins. The potential participants are almost certain to share some assumptions, norms, or rules about conversing, particularly if their cultural and social backgrounds are similar. Very basically, they are likely to take for granted that a two-person conversation will consist of alternative contributions from each person, that only one person will speak at a time and, if through inadequate interaction, regulation, or through interruption, both speakers talk simultaneously, then one or the other should stop very quickly. They may operate with more specific rules of conversation, related, for example, to the social relations between the participants and/or the situation they are interacting in. They may both accept, for instance, that as strangers meeting for the first time, they will participate roughly equally in short alternative contributions, or as interviewer and interviewee, the latter will do most of the talking, or as customer and salesgirl the former will take the initiative in determining the topic of conversation. Such taken-for-granted bases of interaction, usually left implicit rather than made explicit, are amongst the prerequisites for conversation being explored and explicated by micro-sociologists usually dubbed 'ethnomethodologists' (see Douglas, 1970).

But such rules for conversation hardly dictate the very fine-grained 'meshing' that goes on in interaction, and as interaction regulators they are supplemented by communication occurring during the interaction itself. Argyle and Kendon (1967) and Argyle (1969) give accounts of the form that such communication takes, at least in Western societies.

The conversation may be initiated by mutual eye-contact, indicating that the participants are ready and willing to interact. Once the conversation has started, each person looks at the other intermittently. These looks or glances are directed around the other's eyes, last between one and ten seconds each or between 25 and 75 per cent of each person's total time. The amount of time that each spends gazing at the other is considerably more than that spent in mutual eye-contact. The listener is likely to spend more time looking at the speaker than the speaker at the listener. When the speaker, while in full flow, does look at the listener, the latter is likely to nod or give an encouraging vocalization. The speaker, when he starts, probably looks away. When he comes to clear grammatical breaks in what he has to say, the speaker is likely to glance briefly at the listener. When he approaches the end of his contribution he will look longer at the listener. If, however, the speaker hesitates or pauses because he is stuck for a word, or an idea, he is not likely to look at the listener.

Such cues appear to aid conversation regulation in a number of ways. The speaker checks that the listener is in fact still listening, and that he is understanding. A puzzled expression or slight head shake can be enough to tell the speaker to repeat or paraphrase what he has just said. The averting of gaze by the speaker when he stumbles or pauses decreases the likelihood of interruption and mutual talking. The looking up by the speaker just prior to the end of his contribution, signals to the listener that it is almost his turn.

Interpersonal communication

During an encounter a great deal of information is made available regarding the participants and their relations to each other. This information can be organized around three broad topics.

Social and personal identities. If he wishes, a listener or observer can make very many inferences concerning a speaker's background and the social groups to which he belongs, as well as inferences about supposed personality characteristics. The speaker's accent, dress, and even hairstyle might lead to confident assumptions regarding his social class membership and education. Apparently distinctive aspects of the speaker's voice quality, movements, and posture might lead to inferences regarding personality dimensions.

Whether or not these inferences and assumptions are justified is of course a different question and a difficult one to answer. Another difficult problem is that of deciding how much of the available evidence is really communication and how much is merely sign behaviour which can be used for inference making. Suffice it to say that, in addition to inadvertently providing sign behaviour, speakers do communicate information about their social backgrounds and stable personal characteristics via a number of systems of communication. Fuller presentations of material on this topic are given by Robinson (1972) and Argyle (1969).

Temporary states and current attitudes. In addition to inferring or attributing stable characteristics, people also make inferences about temporary states and attitudes. 'Is the person on the other side of the desk really angry with what I've just said?' 'Why should Joe, sitting here drinking beer, seem so anxious?' Such inferences could be based on sign behaviour but, clearly, emotional states can be explicitly communicated. A colleague might tell you that he's angry, or communicate the fact by quite deliberate hand movements or facial expressions. The discussions above of studies by Bugental, Argyle, and others have indicated how non-verbal systems appear to be particularly powerful in this respect.

Social relationships. Interpersonal communication includes not only information about one participant or another but also information regarding the relationship between participants. This can be conveyed non-linguistically. In Western societies, smiling or bodily contact (Jourard, 1966) can very effectively indicate an intimate relationship. A number of other very interesting studies have been carried out on the language of social relationships.

In America, Brown and Ford (1961) explored the use of forms of address in face-to-face interaction with data from various sources, including actual usage in a Boston business firm, usage recorded in a midwestern town, usage in both current and older American plays, and reported usage of business executives from a number of American cities. As would be the case in Britain, they found the most common address forms were first name alone (FN) and title plus last name (TLN). In thinking of when you would call someone Bill rather than Mr Jones, you probably feel it could have something to do with how well you know each other, or again it might be connected with your relative statuses. Brown and Ford showed that, in fact, usage of those address forms, as well as less common ones like last name alone and multiple names, can in large part be predicted from a knowledge of the solidarity or intimacy and the status or power relations of inter-actors. The difference between the mutual use of TLN and the mutual use of FN is a function of intimacy; the non-reciprocal pattern of one person using TLN and the other FN is a function of status differences, with the higher status person receiving the form that is also the more formal, less intimate one. Furthermore, in so far as a dyad progresses from mutual TLN through non-reciprocal usage to mutual FN, it is the higher status person who normally initiates the changes.

In English, a person who is not sure of his status or intimacy relations with another can avoid having to code them by addressing the other as 'you', provided he already has gained the attention of the other person. But speakers of many other languages do not have this option. Even if he does not use FNs or TLNs, a Frenchman has always to choose between using 'tu' or 'vous'. Brown (1965) presents impressive evidence that very similar relations hold amongst status, intimacy, and pronoun forms in a large number of the world's languages as were found with American FN and TLN. Furthermore, the message forms that play a part in the language of social relation-ships are not restricted to forms of address and pronoun use. Brown (1965) and Geertz (1960) amongst others have pointed to the elaborate system of linguistic honorifics that characterize many Far Eastern societies and which also can be shown to vary systematically with status and intimacy relations. And there are probably more aspects of English which systematically correlate with social relations than we sometimes acknowledge. Consider greetings, such as 'hello' as opposed to 'good morning' (see Brown and Ford, 1961) or the use of imperative forms. To whom do you use imperative forms ('Shut the door!'), rather than command with interrogatives ('Could you shut the door?'), or even declaratives ('There's a draught coming in')?

Certainly, I frequently use imperatives to my youngest child but rarely to my wife. And I find that I require a few meetings with someone else's children before I will order them about or threaten them with dire fates in the way I do my own children.

Thus, as far as message forms are concerned, the language of social relations can be very rich. But are status and intimacy the only relevant aspects of the social settings? Somehow, that seems too simple and too tidy. In fact, an obvious question to ask is, what are the bases of status and intimacy? Relative status can be based on a variety of aspects of the relations between two people, as can intimacy. Need status differences based on one's job be coded in exactly the same way as those related to age? Friedrich (1972) has presented a rich and insightful analysis of pronoun usage in nineteenth-century Russia, in which he demonstrates that at least ten components of the social setting could be related to pronominal use. These were: the topic of discourse; the context of the speech event; the age, generation, sex, and kinship status of the participants; dialect; group membership; relative legal and political authority; emotional solidarity. This analysis helps one appreciate that conclusions expressed solely in terms of status and solidarity are broad generalizations, largely justifiable, which ignore many fascinating nuances and fine details.

In conclusion, Friedrich also draws attention to the use of non-linguistic message forms, such as eye-gaze, which may suggest more intimate relations than the verbal forms proclaim. And Brown and Ford (1961) demonstrated that an aspect of kinesics, namely, putting one's hand on someone's shoulder, operated as an index of relationships much as did address forms. Thus, what at first may have seemed like a peculiarity of American FNs and TLNs turns out to be just one manifestation of intricately patterned correspondences between the linguistic (and non-linguistic) forms used by speakers and the social relations that currently hold between them.

Representational communication

Armed with the concepts 'interaction regulation' and 'interpersonal communication' one is still some way from being able to describe a normal conversation, although, at first thought, those two types of communication may seem sufficient to characterize those everyday, banal but important exchanges which the social anthropologist Malinowski (1923) described as 'phatic communion'. With this phrase, he was referring to exchanges of politeness, inquiries about health, comments on the weather, and the like, which, he claimed, fulfilled the primary function of cementing social relationships and for which the exact meaning of the words was largely irrelevant. A very clear instance of this would be the claim, once made to me, at a wedding reception by the father of the groom, that in the receiving line as he smiled and shook hands, he had said to each guest in turn, 'Kippers and jam' and no one appeared to have noticed. Normally however, the meaning and appropriateness of what was said would have a bearing even on such social exchanges. A cheerful extolling of the merits of the weather on a miserable wet day, or a fervent thank you and goodbye on arrival would most probably divert attention from interpersonal matters to the topic of the conversation. Even phatic communion usually involves communication about something over and above social relations.

This third type of communication, representational communication, is what we normally think of when we talk simply of the 'meaning' of what was said. It is the core of linguistic communication, yet it must be admitted it is the most complex of the three types of communication and, in certain respects, the least understood.

A major contribution to understanding it would be the development of an adequate account of the semantics of language (and perhaps of the other systems of communication). 'Semantics', like 'meaning' has been used in a number of different ways, and Lyons (1968) provides a useful introduction to the area. Here the term is being used to refer to the relations between linguistic forms and the extra-linguistic world that they are being applied to. Such an account would entail an analysis of how speakers of a language organize the world around them, an analysis of how they organize the linguistic forms they use, and an account of how the two are related. Think, for example, of what is involved in the differences between breakfast/dinner/ tea, and breakfast/lunch/dinner as accounts of social class differences in eating habits. Referentially or in terms of events, one is indicating in both cases the three major meals of the day, and, to simplify, let us claim that, despite some differences in content and timing, particularly regarding the third meal, the three referents or events are relatively similar for both classes. However, both classes use only two identical terms, 'breakfast' and 'dinner', and in only one case, 'breakfast', is the same meal labelled in the same way by both classes. Obviously, understanding an invitation to dinner should be simpler for two people operating with the same semantic structures than for two people with differences in semantic structures (particularly, in the latter case, if one assumes mutual insensitivity to the differences in each other's backgrounds, that is to very relevant aspects of the social setting).

It must be stressed that, contrary to what might be implied by the simple example above, a semantic analysis involves a great deal more than specifying concrete references for individual words. It involves, for instance, the specification of much more complex semantic relations between sets of persons, objects, and activities and longer linguistic strings. But even if two individuals had, as far as one could tell, identical semantic systems would effective representational communication then be guaranteed? It seems improbable. The mapping of language on to the non-linguistic world is only part of an analysis of representational communication. At least as important would be an understanding of what parts of his semantic system a speaker chooses to use for talking in a particular situation. What does he bother to say? What does he take for granted?

When we talk, we say surprisingly little, at least compared to what we might say to make the same point or compared to what potentially might be relevant. Osgood (1971) has illustrated this very concretely. If a father said to his son, 'Please shut the door' it is most likely (at least in textbook families) that the door would be shut without further ado. Yet if the referential information were to be made completely explicit it could be argued that the father would have had to say something like, 'We both know that you are able to shut doors. There is a door in the far corner of this room. That door is open. I, as your father, desire that that door should be closed by you.' Fortunately, the father like everyone else, would presuppose a great deal and thus would manage with four words rather than thirty-nine.

If representational communication is to be explained as a mixture of semantics and presuppositions, the above example could give the impression that that in turn is a question of analysing the overt message plus the immediate social setting or context. But a further, and final, complication has to be pointed out. Presuppositions can involve factors barely, if at all, represented in either the current social setting or the discourse itself. For example, recently in a case conference one member of a medical team, trying to succinctly convey information about the husband of a patient whose discharge was problematic, resorted to saying, 'Well, he's a typical Rotarian'.

Judging from subsequent comments, this served as a very useful way of transmitting information to half of the clinical team, yet the other half were left mystified. These differences were not a function of differences in understanding at least the dictionary definitions of the words spoken, or of perceptions of prior events in the meeting. Instead they reflected the fact that certain team members shared similar perspectives and assumptions, in this case one might say prejudices, not possessed by the others.

As Rommetweit (1974) has stressed, to understand representational communication one must understand the extent to which two people can build up a shared view of reality, or intersubjectivity. New information is only comprehensible if it can be tied or related to a shared understanding of other information. The presupposed shared reality may be represented in the overt form of an utterance, but often only in a cryptic, minimal way. Thus, to understand what has or has not been communicated, it may be more informative to know what was left unsaid than to know what was actually made explicit. Lengthy and detailed directions can result in thoroughly lost travellers, yet, in the oft-quoted case of Kitty and Levin, in Tolstoy's novel *Anna Karenina*, an exchange of the initial letters of words was sufficient for complete understanding.

Clearly, the appropriateness of the presuppositions made by speaker and listener will prove crucial for representational communication, and this suggests that an analysis of representational communication in terms of presuppositions should not be carried out separately from an analysis of interpersonal communication. What one knows about another person and about one's relation to him is crucial in deciding what to discuss and in determining what is presupposed in discussing it. If social psychology could throw light on the interweaving of social relations and presuppositions it would be much nearer to the heart of communication than it has ever been before.

Communication effectiveness

Since I promised our convenor and editor that I would at least initiate discussion on the vast topic of communication effectiveness, let me close with a few observations on that theme. As is pointed out by Marie Johnston in the next paper, there are at least two views one can take of effectiveness. The more ambitious one is to define it in terms of outcomes, effects, or changes induced by communication, in which case one must immediately raise questions of effectiveness for whom (the doctor, the patient, the health service, the taxpayer) and by what criteria? Is effectiveness to be looked at in terms of task-related outcomes, as is the emphasis in Peter McGuire's paper, or in terms of participants' satisfaction, as in some of Philip Ley's studies? Such problems relating to the consequences of communication are, as yet, beyond the scope of a socio-linguistic analysis, and if there are answers they will have to be found in work within the persuasive communication tradition, to which I briefly alluded at the beginning of this paper and which is the main theme of the last paper by Martin Fishbein.

I shall confine myself to the more limited problem of effectiveness in terms of success or failure in sharing meanings or understandings. What, for example, are the factors which contribute to the receiver ending up with the understanding that the communicator wishes him to have? If I attempted a systematic answer, I would have to go back over my entire analysis because all the bits and pieces are potentially relevant. Mehrabian and Reed (1968) have attempted a detailed review of evidence concerning the components of communication that influence 'communication accuracy', so let me simply point out a few of the links between my analysis and effectiveness as shared understanding.

A number of the concepts I have used appear to have obvious relevance to communication difficulties, when the intended message fails to get through. The difficulty for the sender, the receiver, or both, might be with the overt message being transmitted within one specific system. Alternately, the problem of the message form might be with the interaction of systems, because, for example, the receiver is paying less, or more, attention to certain systems than the sender realizes. There appear to be other communication difficulties which arise from the relationship between the overt message and the immediate social setting. The nature of the participants may not be perceived in the same way by the two parties, as was the case when, as a postgraduate student in psychology who did research in a mental hospital and occasionally wore a white coat, I was once entreated by a worried charge nurse to perform some quite baffling-sounding set of medical acts on a patient who had just collapsed. Or again, the participants may not understand the purpose of the interaction in the same way, one believing the purpose being to exchange information, the other thinking it is to decide on an outcome. Yet again, many failures in communication relate neither to features of the overt message nor to the immediate social setting, but to background presuppositions. The example of the 'typical Rotarian' is one such instance, and it is hard to believe that some of the shortcomings of communication in medical settings are not due to unexamined differences in the backgrounds of doctors and patients.

In addition, the concepts I have discussed can be used to make suggestions about improving effectiveness. One obvious set of possibilities is to increase redundancy within messages. This could be done within one system, or, particularly if time is crucial, one might suggest increasing redundancy across systems, that is using as many systems as possible, provided the communicator is capable of ensuring that he really is transmitting the same message in the different systems. Another suggestion relates to notions of sequential organization, where communicators could often make more use of features, such as explicit sequence signals, which systematically give cohesion to discourse. Yet again, one can at least suggest that attempts be made to minimize the extent to which successful sharing of important meanings is left dependent on participants happening to interpret in the same way fine details of the social context, or fortuitously agreeing on crucial but unchecked presuppositions. To suggest that everything can be made explicit is undoubtedly naïve, but one technique which can help reduce implicitness is the provision of opportunities for feedback, preferably in both directions. It strikes me that, in many situations, a doctor can, if he wishes, interrupt, question, seek further information, and thus try to improve his effectiveness as a receiver by improving the effectiveness of the other person as a sender of information. But does the patient, or for that matter the medical auxiliary, always have adequate opportunities to insist on feedback and thus improve the effectiveness of the doctor as a communicator?

Finally, I hope that my analysis of communication is effective in increasing shared understanding, and that, suitably developed, it might even have implications for outcomes and changes. Meanwhile, I await feedback.

Acknowledgements

Preparation of this paper was aided by SSRC Grant HR 1821. With the permission of the publishers, parts of this paper are taken, in modified and shortened form, from 'Verbal and non-verbal communication', which will appear in H. Tajfel and C. Fraser (eds), *Introducing Social Psychology*, to be published by Penguin Books.

References

ABERCROMBIE, D. (1968). 'Paralanguage', *Br. J. Dis. Commun.* **3**, 55–59.

ARGYLE, M. (1969). *Social Interaction* (London: Methuen).

—— and COOK, M. (1975). *Eye Contact and Mutual Gaze* (Cambridge: Cambridge University Press).

—— and KENDON, A. (1967). 'The experimental analysis of social performance', in Berkowitz, L. (ed.), *Advances in Experimental Social Psychology*, vol. 3 (New York: Academic Press).

—— SALTER, V., NICHOLSON, H., WILLIAMS, M., and BURGESS, P. (1970). 'The communication of inferior and superior attitudes by verbal and non-verbal signals', *Br. J. soc. clin. Psychol.* **9**, 222–31.

BIRDWHISTELL, R. L. (1961). 'Paralanguage twenty-five years after Sapir', in Brosin, H. G. (ed.), *Lectures in Experimental Psychiatry* (Pittsburg: Pittsburg University Press).

—— (1968). 'Kinesics', *International Encyclopedia of the Social Sciences*, **8**, 370–85.

BROWN, R. (1965). *Social Psychology* (Glencoe, Ill.: Free Press).

—— and FORD, M. (1961). 'Address in American English', *J. Abnorm. Soc. Psychol.* **62**, 375–85.

BUGENTAL, D. E., KASWAN, J. M., and LOVE, L. R. (1970). 'Perception of contradictory meanings conveyed by verbal and nonverbal channels', *J. Pers. Soc. Psychol.* **16**, 647–55.

COOK, M. (1971). 'An anatomy of um and er', *New Society*, **17**, no. 455, 577–9.

CRYSTAL, D. (1971). *Linguistics* (Harmondsworth: Penguin).

DOUGLAS, J. D. (ed.) (1970). *Understanding Everyday Life* (New York: Aldine).

EFRON, D. (1941). *Gesture and Environment* (New York: King's Crown).

EKMAN, P., and FRIESEN, W. V. (1969). 'Nonverbal leakage and clues to deception', *Psychiatry*, **32**, 88–106.

FRIEDRICH, P. (1972). 'Social context and semantic feature: The Russian pronominal usage', in Gumperz, J. J., and Hymes, D. (eds), *Directions in Sociolinguistics: The Ethnography of Communication* (New York: Holt, Rinehart & Winston).

GEERTZ, C. (1960). *The Religion of Java* (Glencoe, Ill.: Free Press).

HALLIDAY, M. A. K. (1973). *Explorations in the Functions of Language* (London: Arnold).

HYMES, D. (1972). 'Models of the interaction of language and social life', in Gumperz, J. J., and Hymes, D. (eds), *Directions in Sociolinguistics: The Ethnography of Communication* (New York: Holt, Rinehart & Winston).

JOURARD, S. M. (1966). 'An exploratory study of body accessibility', *Br. J. soc. clin. Psychol.* **5**, 221–31.

LANGACRE, R. W. (1968). *Language and its Structure* (New York: Harcourt, Brace).

LAVER, J. (1968). 'Voice quality and indexical information', *Br. J. Dis. Commun.* **3**, 43–54.

—— and HUTCHESON, S. (eds) (1972). *Communication in Face-to-Face Interaction* (Harmondsworth: Penguin).

LEACH, E. (1972). 'The influence of cultural context on non-verbal communication in man', in Hinde, R. A. (ed.), *Non-Verbal Communication* (Cambridge: Cambridge University Press).

LYONS, J. (1968). *Introduction to Theoretical Linguistics* (Cambridge: Cambridge University Press).

MALINOWSKI, S. (1923). 'The problem of meaning in primitive languages', Supplement to Ogden, C. K., and Richards, I. A., *The Meaning of Meaning* (London: Routledge and Kegan Paul).

McGUIRE, W. J. (1968). 'The nature of attitudes and attitude change', in Lindzey, G., and Aronson, E. (eds), *Handbook of Social Psychology*, 2nd edn, vol. 3 (Reading, Mass.: Addison-Wesley).

MEHRABIAN, A., and REED, H. (1968). 'Some determinants of communication accuracy', *Psychol. Bull.* 70, 365–81.

MOSCOVICI, S. (1967). 'Communication processes and the properties of language', in Berkowitz, L. (ed.), *Advances in Experimental Social Psychology*, vol. 3 (New York: Academic Press).

OSGOOD, C. E. (1971). 'Where do sentences come from?' in Steinberg, D. D., and Jakobovits, L. A. (eds), *Semantics: An Interdisciplinary Reader* (Cambridge: Cambridge University Press).

ROBINSON, W. P. (1972). *Language and Social Behaviour* (Harmondsworth: Penguin).

ROMMETWEIT, R. (1974). *On Message Structure: A Framework for the Study of Language and Communication* (London: Wiley).

SHEFLEN, A. E. (1964). 'The significance of posture in communication systems', *Psychiatry*, 27, 316–31.

SINCLAIR, J. M., and COULTHARD, R. M. (1975). *Towards an Analysis of Discourse* (Oxford: Oxford University Press).

VINE, I. (1969). 'Communication by facial-visual signals', in Crook, J. H. (ed.), *Social Behaviour in Animals and Man* (London: Academic Press).

Communication of patients' feelings in hospital

Marie Johnston

Research Officer
Health Services Evaluation Group
Department of the Regius Professor of Medicine
University of Oxford

Communication of patients' feelings in hospital

This paper considers the measurement of communication focusing on the problem of assessing whether communication has occurred. For any communication to occur, there must be a sender and a receiver and a message passing between the two. The process may fail at various points; the sender may not output the message or he may output it in a way that is unintelligible to the receiver; the receiver may fail to input the message or he may interpret the message wrongly; or the message may be interrupted or distorted in its passage from sender to receiver. The similarity between the message as the sender recognizes it and the message as the receiver perceives it indicates the success of communication *per se*.

Examining the literature on communication between patients and health service professionals, three gaps are discernible and these concern the criterion, content, and direction of communication respectively. First, the criteria of success usually go beyond assessing whether communication has been achieved and examine whether the communication has been successful in reaching some further target. For example, the target is often to influence the behaviour of the receiver, as when the doctor recommends a procedure to a patient, and there are a number of studies (reviewed by Blackwell, 1973) in which the success of communication is indicated by the patient's compliance with doctor's instructions. In other studies the criterion of effective communication is the receiver's satisfaction with communications. It is obviously important to examine such variables, as communication would be a trivial consideration if it achieved nothing. However, frequently the conclusion is that communication has been a failure by the criteria used and it is not clear whether communication has occurred and has been unsuccessful, or has not occurred. There are a few studies which have used mismatch between what was sent and what the receiver reports as their measure of outcome. For example, Ley and Spelman (1965) have done a number of studies in which the criterion is the amount of information the patient can remember from a set which the doctor is known to have given. Joyce *et al.* (1969) have also presented work of this kind.

These studies hint at a second gap which exists. The most readily examined communications are those in which the message is (*a*) a statement of fact and (*b*) intentionally delivered. As a result, there is little information about the communication of thoughts, feelings, opinions, etc., or messages which are delivered incidentally, in parallel to the main content of the communication. One might argue that such communications are of little importance in medicine and that it is basically statements of fact which count. However, there is evidence that the more ambiguous, emotional messages also play a critical part in determining the effectiveness of communication. Freemon *et al.* (1971) used a modified Bales's interaction analysis to categorize statements in various ways, including the nature of the effect expressed. In general, they found that the expression of positive effect, that is being nice, is associated with greater satisfaction and compliance in the patients. While they also found that information giving affects the outcome variables, this study does illustrate the importance of the more ambiguous, affective, messages in medical communications. Such messages are clearly important in communications from doctor to patient but are perhaps even more important in communication from patient to doctor. For example, communication of pain falls within this category and is clearly of importance. However, as Bond (1970) has demonstrated, perception of patients' pain is not directly related to the pain the patient experiences.

This leads to the final gap to be considered which concerns the direction of the communication. In most studies, the sender is the doctor, the receiver the patient. Apart from some work on the failure of patients to consult their doctor, that is the failure of the patient to become the sender of a message, there has been little research on the transmission of messages in the direction patient to health-care professional. It seems self-evident that these are also important and the dearth of such studies is probably due to the difficulty of controlling or assessing what message the patient is sending.

Broadly, the aim of this research was to examine the success with which non-factual messages passed from patients to health-care professionals. Within this context, the aim was to look at differences in the pattern of communication of physical and psychological feelings. Baer *et al.* (1970) have demonstrated that nurses are more likely to infer pain from verbal, spoken messages, while they are more likely to infer psychological distress from non-verbal messages. It is possible that patients use the separate communication channels in a similar manner, communicating the pain verbally and distress non-verbally. A mismatch between the patients' use of the channels and the nurses' methods of inference would certainly lead to failures of communication. It is clearly possible that there might be a different pattern of communication of pain and psychological distress. This study extends the comparison to include other forms of physical problems, in addition to pain.

The basic technique used was to present patients with questionnaires to describe their feelings and simultaneously to ask one nurse to complete similar forms for each patient. In this way, the state of the messages was measured at the sender, patient, end of the communication and at the receiver, nurse, end and the correspondence between these two taken as the outcome.

Method

The research worker went to the wards involved in the study intermittently to avoid any systematic bias which might result from regular visits. Every patient who fitted the description below was asked to fill in questionnaires. The patient was instructed to complete the forms to show how she felt at that moment. As nearly simultaneously as possible, a nurse was asked to complete a similar form for that patient, to describe how the patient felt.

The nurses were told that it was a study of the extent to which patients revealed their feelings to nurses and that the patient was completing the form to describe how she felt. There was no possibility of contact between the nurse and patient after instructions, before completing the form. In allocating patients to nurses, each nurse on any ward was given a similar number of patients on each occasion. Within these limits, allocation was random, but the nurses were permitted to exchange patients if they did not know the ones they had been allocated. This procedure was adopted so that no single nurse was overburdened by the study and that deviations from randomness should maximize the degree of communication.

Subjects

The study was conducted in three gynaecology wards. The patients were all post-operative, on average four days after operation, range

1 to 17. The nurses were all day nurses, on duty when the research worker called. Forty-eight patients and nineteen nurses took part.

Questionnaires

The Hospital Adjustment Inventory (HAI) (De Wolfe *et al.*, 1966) was used as a measure of psychological distress. Each of the twenty-two items asks about a different worry and the patient is required to give a YES/NO answer. Table 1 presents a sample of the items, the first three items being frequently endorsed, the final three items being infrequently endorsed in the current study.

Physical feelings were examined using the Recovery Inventory (RI) (Wolfer and Davis, 1970) which contains eight items related to physical welfare (sleep, appetite, strength and energy, stomach condition, bowel condition, ability to urinate, ability to do things for self, ability to move around and get out of bed by self) and one psychological item, 'interest in surroundings', in addition to two items on pain, one relating to duration, one to intensity. The first nine items were rated on six-point scales from 'very poor' to 'excellent' while the pain items also had six-point scales, from 'none' to 'very much' and 'very mild to 'extremely intense'.

The Hospital Adjustment Inventory preceded the Recovery Inventory and nurses and patients were presented with forms which were identical except for a space for the nurse's identification.

Table 1. *Sample of Hospital Adjustment Inventory items.*

10. Do you worry about being transferred to another ward or hospital?

11. Do you wonder whether you are making as much progress in recovering from your illness as you should be making?

21. Do you worry about illness or possible illness in your family?

 4. Does it bother you to have to associate so closely with people on the ward?

16. Are you afraid that your husband may walk out on you while you are in the hospital?

18. Do you wonder whether you will be accepted by people after you leave the hospital?

Results

Both questionnaires were scored so that the patients' scores increased
with worsening state; thus on the HAI a high score indicates many
worries, on the RI an item scoring high was very poor or indicated
more pain.

Perception of psychological and physical distress

The mean scores of nurses and patients are shown in Table 2. On the
HAI, nurses have significantly higher scores than patients, indicating
that they perceive the patients to have more worries than the patients
report. On the RI however, the nurses tend to have lower scores,
significantly lower on appetite, strength and energy, pain duration,
and pain intensity. Table 2 also shows the number of patients for
whom the nurses over- or under-estimate the patients' assessments

Table 2. *Discrepancy between nurses' and patients' responses*

	Mean scores		Nurse errors	
	Patients	*Nurses*	*Over- estimates*	*Under- estimates*
HOSPITAL ADJUSTMENT				
INVENTORY	3·41	9·08†	42	3*
RECOVERY INVENTORY				
Sleep	2·47	2·43	17	18
Appetite	3·07	2·56†	8	23*
Strength	2·92	2·53*	7	21*
Stomach condition	2·05	2·18	16	15
Bowel condition	2·98	2·72	10	18
Ability to urinate	2·03	1·91	14	16
Independence	2·16	2·00	13	20
Mobility	2·09	2·14	13	14
Interest	1·57	1·94	24	11*
Pain—Duration	3·04	2·57*	11	24*
Pain—Intensity	3·23	2·47†	7	27*

* Statistically significant differences between nurses' and patients' mean scores
or number of over- and under-estimates.
† $p < 0.05$. $p < 0.01$.

for each score. Nurses significantly over-estimate psychological distress as shown by the HAI and the RI item 'interest in surroundings'. On all the physical state items except 'stomach condition', the nurses under-estimate the problem compared with the patients; this is significant for 'appetite' and 'strength' and for both the pain ratings.

From these data, it is clear that nurses overestimate psychological problems and underestimate physical problems compared with patients. This gives considerable support to the hypothesis that there are differences in the patterns of communication of pain and psychological distress.

Nurse–patient communication

As a first step in the analysis of nurse–patient communication, one can say that certain systematic biases are apparent. However, this only covers the general level of communication, that is what nurses generally believe about patients generally and it is important to investigate the success of the communications at a one-to-one level. If one assumes for this analysis that the patients report their feelings accurately, then nurses can give a correct response, that is one identical to the patient's, in three ways. The first is by pure chance. Secondly, by a general knowledge of what patients think and feel they can predict to the individual patient; the more information that is available about the patient, the more accurate this prediction is likely to be. Thirdly, the nurse can predict the patient's response accurately by specific knowledge of what the individual patient thinks and feels.

In examining the specific communication success, it is essential to make some allowance for the over-all responding rate of both patients and nurses. Otherwise, for example on the HAI, there would be a high failure rate due to the over-all bias in responding noted in the initial analysis.

Hospital Adjustment Inventory

The first question is whether the proportion of correct responses by nurses exceeds chance expectations. Basically one is asking 'Does one-to-one communication exist?' The average percentage of correct judgements per nurse–patient pair is 64 per cent. In order to examine whether this significantly exceeds the chance level of 50 per cent, the phi coefficient of correlation (Garrett, 1962) was used to estimate the degree of association between the nurses' and patients' judgements.

First, phi was calculated for each nurse–patient pair and the values ranged from $+0.69$ to -0.67. On the whole, the correlations are positive, the distribution over all 48 being 35 positive, 7 negative, and 6 zero. Thus there are significantly more positive than negative correlations, indicating a clear association between nurses' and patients' judgements. However, evidence of a significant positive association between the nurse and patient's ratings is found in only thirteen pairs and in two pairs there is a significant negative association. It would appear that, although there is evidence of communication over-all, a significant level of communication is achieved in a limited number of cases. These cases will be discussed again later.

Secondly, the phi coefficient was calculated for each of the 22 items and here the values ranged from $+0.42$ to -0.15. There were 11 positive, 7 negative, and 4 zero coefficients and thus no evidence of a positive association between nurses' and patients' judgements. Only three items exceed the 0.05 level of significance:

'Do you worry whether visitors will come to see you?'

'Do you worry about whether you will get a pension or compensation?'

'Do you worry about whether your children are being cared for properly while you are in hospital?'

To summarize, considered over-all, nurses perform at better than chance level, in predicting worries for individual patients, but when one considers individual nurse–patient pairs significant prediction is seldom achieved. They are not successful at predicting which patients worry about each item.

However, it is still possible that relative accuracy was achieved, nurses achieving the same *pattern* of results as patients. This was examined by correlating the patient's number of worries with the number estimated by the nurse, over patients; the correlation was 0.23 which, with 46 degrees of freedom, is not significant at the 0.05 level. Fig. 1 shows the frequency of YES responses for each nurse and patient and clearly there is no relationship between the two patterns. The nurses' tendency to get higher scores than patients is apparent. These results suggest that the nurses cannot predict which patients have most worries.

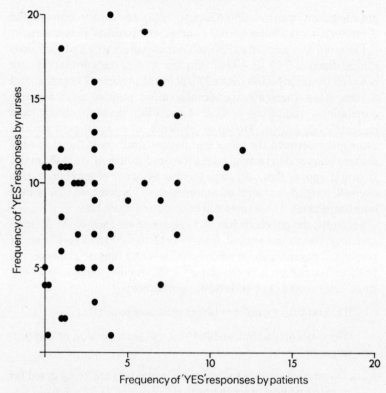

Fig. 1. *HAI: frequency of YES responses by nurses and patients plotted by nurse–patient pairs.*

They may, however, be able to predict which worries patients have. This is a question about the nurses' general knowledge of patients, not the knowledge about individual patients. Fig. 2 shows the frequency of nurses' and patients' YESs for each item. Again the higher scores of the nurses is clear, but the nurses' scores follow a similar pattern to the patients'. The correlation between nurses' and patients' scores over items is 0·82, indicating that nurses can estimate what patients are most likely to be worried about.

The ability to predict which items patients worry about most might contribute to the success of the one-to-one communication where it exists, that is in the 13 nurse–patient pairs for whom the phi coefficient was significant. It is possible that these 13 patients produce patterns of judgements which are close to the average and would therefore be

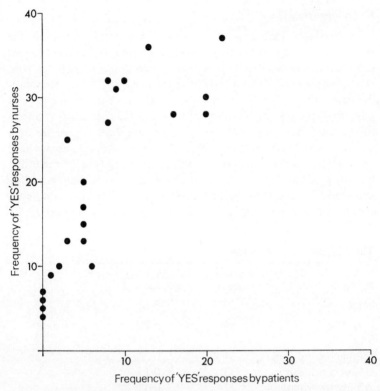

Fig. 2. *HAI: frequency of YES responses by nurses and patients plotted by items.*

predictable from a general knowledge of patients. In all, 23 patients make judgements which correlate (point-biserial) with the average over-all patients positively and significantly; of these, 10 belong to the group of 13 showing significant association with the nurse's judgements. Thus there is a significant tendency ($\chi^2 = 4 \cdot 52$, $p < 0 \cdot 05$) for these patients who show significant communication to be producing typical response patterns which might be predictible from general knowledge of patients.

It appears that although nurses know *what* patients worry about, they cannot tell *which patients* do most worrying, nor even *how many* worries patients have. For some patients they can predict what the patient worries about, but at least some part of this is due to their success in predicting the performance of average patients.

Recovery Inventory

It is probably inappropriate to consider over-all scores on the Recovery Inventory as was done for the Hospital Adjustment Inventory because of the diversity of items; therefore the items are considered separately. Table 3 shows the percentage of correct responses for each item on the RI, ranging from 17 per cent on 'intensity of pain' to 40 per cent on 'mobility'. Examining the data using χ^2 allows for the frequency of use of the response categories. There are only two significant deviations from chance. In one 'mobility', nurses have more correct answers than one would expect by chance. In the other, 'intensity of pain', they have fewer correct answers than would be expected by chance. While this latter result is difficult to interpret, the combined results demonstrate rather poor communication.

Table 3. *Recovery Inventory results*

Item	Percentage correct	Correlation between nurses and patients
Sleep	26	0·13
Appetite	34	0·29*
Strength	35	0·09
Stomach condition	31	0·22
Bowel condition	33	0·19
Ability to urinate	27	0·43†
Independence	28	0·07
Mobility	40†	0·26*
Interest	24	0·24*
Pain—duration	26	0·14
Pain—intensity	17*	0·08

*$p < 0.05$.   †$p < 0.01$.

As with the HAI, one can use correlations to see if nurses and patients have similar patterns despite the lack of absolute accuracy. The correlations between nurses' and patients' responses for each item are shown in the final column of Table 3. They are generally low, with only four significant, 'appetite', 'ability to urinate', 'mobility', and 'interest in surroundings'. One must conclude that nurses and patients do not communicate this kind of information efficiently.

Discussion

In summary, these results suggest that the communication about feelings between nurses and patients is very limited at the one-to-one level. While there is some evidence of significant communication of psychological problems, only one of the physical items showed significant evidence of communication and indeed one item gave poorer than chance prediction. Further evidence of a difference between communication of physical and psychological problems is given in the tendency of the nurses to overestimate psychological problems and underestimate physical problems.

These data lead one to examine why communication was so unsuccessful rather than to dissect the components of success. It may be unsuccessful because it was quite an extreme test of communication. The patient may or may not wish or attempt to communicate the messages being examined, although she may output the messages unintentionally. Even if the patient wishes to output them, she may do so inefficiently. She may even attempt an indirect communication, for example, via another patient, which may be distorted or lost en route. The nurse may not present the opportunity for the communication, or she may fail to recognize that the patient is sending a message or she may misunderstand the message.

Perhaps this type of communication is bad because it is irrelevant to the requirements of the situation. One might argue that it is not necessary for the nurse to know which aspects of their home lives worry patients in order for them to perform their nursing duties adequately. On the other hand, surely the nurses must be making some estimate of how much pain each patient suffers, if only to administer analgesics; the data would suggest that nurses do so badly on assessment of pain that analgesics might more reliably be given to patients in greatest pain by distributing them randomly, nurses performing worse than chance. This may explain Bond's (1970) finding that administration of analgesics bears no clear relationship to patients' reports of pain. One might also have expected that nurses would know who were most worried if only to seek to secure relief for these patients; in so far as number of worries is indicative of patients' over-all anxiety level, nurses fail on this criterion too.

A possible explanation of the poor communication may lie in the responder's interpretation of what was required on the questionnaires. For example, patients might operate a stricter criterion before they admitted to worries believing that they were only meant to check items on which they worried more than the average patient. Such a performance might explain the excess of worries reported by the nurses. However, one would have to postulate an opposite bias on the RI to explain the excess of problems in the patients' data and it seems improbable that the strict criterion would not be maintained throughout.

More generally, one might suggest that the limited level of apparent communication arises because patients do not admit how they feel on these tests. However, for the Recovery Inventory, one can point to the validity of the test which shows that patients' scores change in parallel with other indicators of recovery; it is unlikely that such validity would be obtained if the patients were adopting untruthful response strategies. One cannot make the same claims for the validity of the Hospital Adjustment Inventory, but it is perhaps less necessary here as some evidence of communication was found.

Finally, one might wish to ask how important are such communications. The results of this study suggest that nurses are not very aware of patients' worries and, therefore, probably inaccurate in their assessments of the type of information patients require. As a result, one might expect that any attempts to improve communications would be doomed to failure unless there was some improvement in the selection of the appropriate areas for such increased efforts. This is borne out indirectly by Houghton's (1968) study in which attempts were made to improve as many aspects of communications as possible, but the results showed no increase in patient satisfaction. Such failures are important when one considers that communications is the aspect of hospital care which patients are most likely to criticize and over-all patient satisfaction is largely determined by their satisfaction with communications. It is possible that the ability to identify which problems cause worry and require information is essential to improving patients' satisfaction with communication and, perhaps, over-all satisfaction with their hospital care.

References

BAER, E., DAVITZ, L. J., and LIEB, R. (1970). 'Inference of physical pain and psychological distress 1: in relation to verbal and nonverbal patient communication', *Nursing Research*, **19**, 388–92.

BLACKWELL, B. (1973). 'Drug therapy: Patient compliance', *New Engl. J. Med.* **289**, 249–52.

BOND, M. R. (1970). 'Psychological aspects of pain', PhD thesis (Sheffield University).

DE WOLFE, A. S., BARRELL, R. P., and CUMMINGS, J. W. (1966). 'Patient variables in emotional response to hospitalization for physical illness', *J. Consult. Psychol.* **30**, 68–72.

FREEMON, B., NEGRETE, V. F., DAVIS, M., and KORSCH, B. M. (1971). 'Gaps in doctor–patient communication: doctor–patient interaction analysis', *Pediat. Res.* **5**, 298–311.

GARRETT, H. E. (1962). *Statistics in Psychology and Education*, 5th edn (London: Longmans).

HOUGHTON, H. (1968). 'Problems of hospital communication: an experimental study', in McLachlan, G. (ed.), *Problems and Progress in Medical Care*, Third Series (Oxford University Press for the Nuffield Provincial Hospitals Trust).

JOYCE, C. R. B., CAPLE, G., MASON, M., REYNOLDS, E., and MATHEWS, J. A. (1969). 'Quantitative study of doctor–patient communication', *Q. Jl Med.* **38**, 183–94.

WOLFER, J. A., and DAVIS, C. E. (1970). 'Assessment of surgical patients' pre-operative emotional condition and post-operative welfare', *Nursing Research*, **19**, 402–14.

Training medical students to communicate

The development and evaluation of an interviewing model and training procedure

Peter Maguire

Senior Lecturer
Department of Psychiatry
University of Manchester
(*Formerly Clinical Tutor in Psychiatry*
University of Oxford)

Derek Rutter

Lecturer in Psychology
University of Warwick
(*Formerly Research Psychologist*
Department of Psychiatry
University of Oxford)

Training medical students to communicate

Much of the communication which occurs between doctors and patients concerns the gathering of information about the patient and his problems. Hence, it is essential that medical students become skilled at eliciting such data and at fostering the trust which is necessary if patients are to comply with advice and treatment. Unfortunately, there is now considerable evidence that medical training is failing to equip students with these basic interviewing skills. The purpose of this paper is to review this evidence, describe an interviewing model and training procedure which have been designed to help medical students improve their interviewing skills, and discuss the results of their use.

Deficiencies in interviewing techniques

The evidence derives from two groups of studies: those in which medical student interviews have been observed directly, and those which have monitored clinical practice.

Direct observation of medical student interviews

When bedside interviews by twenty-one medical students were observed during an introductory medical clerkship (Hinz, 1966), it was noted that the students were particularly poor at obtaining a history of the present illness and frequently omitted to explore relevant social and psychological aspects of their patients' illnesses. Despite the two months devoted to the course, two-thirds of the students found the history-taking procedure difficult to master. Hinz attributed these interviewing difficulties to the students' inexperience and lack of clinical knowledge. However, analyses of audiotape (Tapia, 1972) and videotape recordings (Anderson *et al.*, 1970) of interviews conducted by similarly inexperienced students with general medical and surgical patients suggested that these difficulties were as much due to a lack of important interview skills as to mere ignorance of clinical facts. Although it would have been comforting to claim that medical students developed the necessary interviewing skills as a result of their later clinical training, our own preliminary observations suggested that these improvements usually failed to take place. We sought to confirm this by a detailed analysis of interviews conducted by more senior medical students during a psychiatric clerkship.

Fifty students were each asked to interview a psychiatric patient previously unknown to them in order to obtain a history of the present illness or problems. The students were told that the purpose of the interview was to provide a baseline for assessing their interviewing skills. They were informed that they had fifteen minutes for their interview, were to concentrate on finding out about current problems, were to be responsible for ending the interview on time, and would be required to write up a careful history afterwards. The fifteen-minute limit was chosen because it approximated much more closely to the time they would have for their interviews when qualified, than the hour or more they were usually allowed.

Patients were selected according to several criteria: all were recovering from one of two very common types of psychiatric disorder (either depressive illness or anxiety neurosis), were thought likely to co-operate well with the students, had initially presented with complaints suggestive of organic pathology or had concurrent physical illnesses. It was intended that the test situation should draw upon basic interviewing skills rather than the more sophisticated behaviours required to cope with, for example, garrulous, demanding, reticent, or hostile patients. The interviews were recorded on videotape and the students' interviewing behaviours analysed.

The major finding was that these more senior medical students displayed exactly the same lack of interviewing skills as those much less experienced students. The study confirmed that students who were close to their final examinations performed no better than students with less clinical experience.

Their deficiences in interviewing skills were shown in the following ways.

A paucity of information obtained. A major function of the history-taking interview is to obtain as much relevant and accurate information as possible within the time available. It was, therefore, alarming to discover how little information was obtained. The students reported a median of only fourteen items of 'acceptable' information in their written histories. This represented only a quarter of those facts which were judged independently to be easily obtainable in the time available. As in the histories taken by introductory course students, relevant psychological and social aspects of the patient's problems were most commonly neglected. A third of the students even failed to elicit the patient's main illness or problems. When told of this low efficiency in data gathering, most of the students were very surprised, for they had seriously over-estimated the amount of useful information they had obtained.

Failure to control the interview. Much of the students' inefficiency in data-gathering seemed to derive from their inability to keep patients to the point. All too often, they allowed the patients to talk at length of matters quite unrelated to their present problems. The students did not appear to know how or when to interrupt and redirect them to more relevant topics. Moreover, their difficulties in controlling the interview sometimes had other negative effects. For example, when some students realized that the information they were being given was irrelevant, but did not know how to interrupt, they became frustrated. They communicated their feelings to the patient by look-ing bored and becoming restless. In consequence, their patients ceased to co-operate, and the students were left feeling even more uncertain about what to do next.

The students were acutely aware of this problem of control but were afraid that any attempts to interrupt and redirect the conversa-tion would make the patients unco-operative and resentful. Yet the patients had been chosen because they were co-operative and it was evident that when students did try to redirect them, the patients were only too willing to try and give the interviewers the data they wanted. The students also reported that they found the time limit particularly difficult to cope with. Only 10 per cent ended their interviews on time. They attributed this to two factors; they were normally allowed at least forty-five minutes to one hour to take a history and so had never had to resolve the problems posed by a more limited time period; they also thought that looking at their watches or a clock would be interpreted by the patients as a lack of concern. The students readily admitted that they had given little thought to the amount of time they would have for interviewing once they qualified.

Lack of a systematic interview procedure. Very few students appeared
to follow any predictable sequence of questions, apart from those
directed at a review of the major physical systems of the body. Nor
was it possible to discern any consistency in the way they began,
conducted, or terminated their interviews. There was often no
obvious logical connection between consecutive topics. As a result
there were often crucial gaps in the histories they obtained and
recorded. Unfortunately, it frequently seemed a matter of chance
which areas they covered. This applied particularly to whether they
tried to find out how the illness or key problems had affected the
patient and his family, the treatments already given to the patient for
the present illness, and the presence of practical, psychological, and
social problems.

The students attributed this lack of any definite procedure to the
fact that, during their clinical training, they had not received any
detailed guidance about how to conduct interviews. They claimed
they had been given little more than a list of questions which should
be asked routinely of physically ill patients.

Premature and restricted focus. Another interviewing difficulty concerned the mental set which the students appeared to have about the
types of problems most patients would complain of. They generally
assumed that patients would have only one main problem and that
this was much more likely to be organic than psychological or social
in nature. Hence, the students tended to probe no further than the
first problem volunteered by the patient, particularly when it was
organic in type.

This usually resulted in their failing to elicit other important
problems. Students' preferences for a single pathology and for organic
illness were strengthened by their reluctance to ask any questions
about their patients' personal lives, especially their marriages, other
key personal relationships, social life, sexual adjustment, and mood.
When these topics were raised spontaneously by the patients, the
students tried to gloss over them and so avoid any further inquiry.
When students broached these topics themselves they often did so in
a very hesitant and embarrassed manner. They explained that their
diffidence about touching on more personal areas of inquiry was due
to their anxiety that patients found such questions unacceptable and
intrusive. Yet when students did cover these areas, all the patients
gave helpful responses.

Lack of clarification. Even when relevant information was successfully obtained, it was often confused and contradictory. This was partly due to students' reluctance to ask patients for clarification. For example, when one particular patient complained that his main problem had been 'confusion', the student took this to mean an organic brain syndrome. He subsequently asked only questions which related to that possibility. Yet the patient had wanted to explain that by 'confusion' he meant that he had felt slowed down, become very low in spirits, and unable to concentrate. The uncertainty of much of the information was also due to students' failure to detect or confront patients with obvious inconsistencies in their accounts. None of the students had any routine way of cross-checking the accuracy of the story they had obtained with the patient, or of ensuring that they had elicited all the main problems before the interview ended.

Lack of precision. The students' willingness to accept data that were extremely vague was a further obstacle to eliciting firm and consistent information. Although accurate dating of important events and of the times of onset of key problems is crucial to a consideration of possible aetiological relationships, few students made any effort to encourage patients to date their experiences accurately. They were equally imprecise when they covered current treatments, and it was rare for the exact drugs, their doses, clinical and unwanted effects to be firmly established, even though the patients frequently possessed the necessary information, or had the appropriate bottles of tablets in a coat pocket or handbag.

Unresponsiveness to verbal and non-verbal cues. Most patients provided helpful verbal cues about their main problems. However, these were not often noticed or responded to by the students. For example, one particular patient complained initially that his main worry was his dizzy spells. He went on to say that he had been admitted to hospital because these had failed to abate and had made him feel 'very low'. Although he made reference to this mood change five more times within the first eight minutes of the interview, the student concerned did not notice this. As a result he failed to realize that the patient's main problem was not the dizzy spells but a depressive illness whose onset had preceded these spells by three months. Interestingly the student's behaviour paralleled what had happened in real life. This patient had been subjected repeatedly to physical investigation before it was eventually realized that his main problem was depression. He later responded very well to anti-depressant treatment. Similar in-attention extended to non-verbal cues, even when these were gross. For example, when one patient was finding it difficult to recall an important sequence of events, she reached down to her handbag and began to take out a diary in which she had recorded details of her illness. The student missed this. Yet, had he responded appropriately the diary would have given him an accurate, vivid, and rapid summary of her problems. This unresponsiveness was most noticeable when patients gave cues suggestive of emotional upset. When patients became tearful, irritable, or anxious, the students usually tried to encourage the patient to move on to a neutral topic. They subsequently indicated that they did this because they feared that if they responded to such cues they would precipitate even more distress, a possibility they felt ill-trained to handle, and because it made them feel very uneasy.

Deficiencies in question style. Most of the inquiries that students made were in the form of leading questions. This question style biased and restricted the data they obtained and led to a loss of important information. The students also commonly asked several questions at once. This made it difficult for the patients to remember and respond to each element in the questions. For example, one student, inquiring about the possibility of depressive symptoms asked 'you were losing weight? and what about sleeping? . . . you weren't getting off?, waking early? . . . I mean how did this all affect you?' The patient responded by saying 'I was sleeping badly'. The student did not repeat any of the other elements of his question.

Failure to prepare the patient. Only a fifth of the students explained exactly who they were, their status, or whom they were currently working with. It was almost as uncommon for them to explain their intentions, or to ensure that the patient was at ease, before they asked questions. The majority immediately rushed into asking questions about the main complaints. However, the patients said after their interviews that they wished doctors would make more effort to explain the kinds of information they required, the procedure they intended to follow and the time they had available. They suggested that knowledge of this information would encourage them to com-municate the more essential problems, or allow them to discuss with the doctor a time period that would be more appropriate to their needs.

Lack of self-awareness. Some students displayed mannerisms which seriously hampered their attempts to relate to their patients. One student repeatedly answered 'yes' to a patient in so bored a manner that the patient was reduced to silence. Another adopted an extremely casual and sprawling posture. The patient interpreted this as indifference and gave little further information in the interview. While both students stated that their behaviours were part of their usual interview styles, neither had been aware that their mannerisms had such negative consequences.

Note-taking and accuracy of the students' case-histories. Most students found it difficult both to take notes and look at the patient. They were often seen to be still busy writing, with their heads bent over their notes, when the patient looked up for some sign of attention. Despite the time ostensibly spent writing detailed notes, some of the histories written up after the interviews contained only a small proportion of the information elicited during the interview. However, when students elected not to take notes, their omissions were even greater.

This study of fifty medical students therefore revealed serious deficiencies in their interviewing skills, and it is important to stress at this point that most of the students accepted that the test situation reflected accurately their everyday interviewing difficulties. Only a few students argued that their deficiences had been due entirely to the stress of the test interview. Moreover, audiotape interviews conducted by twelve of the same students with new patients in a psychiatric out-patient clinic revealed no higher level of skill than the test interviews. We considered it reasonable to conclude that the problems revealed were genuine, and that their medical training was failing to equip these students with basic interviewing skills.

Strong support for our view came from the work of Helfer (1970). In a videotape study at the University of Colorado, he asked sixty senior medical students to interview simulated parents of sick children. He found that they used interviewing techniques which hampered the collection of relevant information. He also noted that they commonly asked leading questions, used unfamiliar medical terminology, cut off the patients' communications, failed to ask questions about important interpersonal aspects of the cases, and rarely gave any feedback or reassurance. He suggested that medical training had eroded these students' innate interpersonal skills. He sought to test this hypothesis by a comparison of senior medical students with freshmen. He found that senior medical students interviewed significantly less well. They obtained less information about important personal problems, failed more often to elicit other key difficulties and asked leading questions more frequently than the freshmen students.

In view of the nature and extent of these deficiences, it is perhaps of some consolation that medical students are well aware of their lack of certain basic interviewing skills (MacNamara, 1974). They report that they have most difficulty talking to patients about their marriages, taking a sexual history, dealing with silences, and complain that they do not know how to ask questions, facilitate helpful responses, or provide reassurance.

Studies of clinical practice

Monitoring of clinical practice has shown that qualified doctors display similar interviewing difficulties. In a valuable study carried out in the Los Angeles Children's Hospital, the visits to a paediatric out-patient clinic of 800 mothers and their children were monitored by means of audiotape recordings (Korsch *et al.*, 1968). It was found that in over two-thirds of cases, the paediatricians failed to elicit the mothers' main concerns about their children and their expectations about diagnosis and treatment. They seldom realized the extent to which mothers blamed themselves for their children's illnesses, and most of the mothers' questions went unheeded. This unresponsiveness of the paediatricians led, in some instances, to the women ceasing to try to give any further information. It was also evident that when doctors were insensitive in this way, their subsequent advice was much less likely to be registered by the women.

It was further found that the doctors used difficult and unfamiliar technical language in over half their interviews, and commonly failed to introduce themselves by name. They usually paid scant attention to the possible adverse influence of external factors on the mothers. For example, they were often unaware that the mothers had been upset by a long wait in the clinic, by the lack of privacy, the risk of interruptions, or preoccupation with practical matters such as the welfare of other children left at home. Another crucial finding concerned the issue of time. For, although many of these paediatricians might have been tempted to argue that their problems were solely due to their having insufficient time in busy clinics to interview more effectively, Korsch and her co-authors could find no relationship between the time the paediatricians spent and the quality of their interviews. Indeed, they commented that much valuable time was lost through 'ineffective verbalization' on the part of the doctors who were, for example, often trapped into unhelpful arguments with the mothers. The authors concluded that it was not the amount of time that was crucial, but the way the available time was used. They suggested that a short period spent at the beginning of an interview in establishing the patient's main concerns and expectations would save a great deal of time later and make for a more satisfactory doctor–patient relationship.

The difficulties these doctors appeared to have in eliciting certain of their patients' main problems, particularly when these were psychological or social in nature, were also noted in a study of 230 consecutive admissions to two general medical wards (Maguire *et al.*, 1974). Of the 23 per cent of patients shown by independent psychiatric interview to be suffering from definite psychiatric illness, the psychiatric problems had been detected in just under a half. This failure to detect important psychological problems, particularly depressive illness, appeared related to the interviewing techniques of the house physicians, and their almost exclusive preoccupation with the physical well-being of their patients. They failed to ask routinely about mood or psychological responses to illness, and said this was due to their reluctance to inquire closely about these matters, particularly if the patients were suffering from malignant disease. While their physical orientation was understandable since they were serving an acutely ill population, it nevertheless resulted in the neglect of other major problems.

Other evidence has indicated that even when a doctor possesses an appropriate repertoire of interviewing strategies and techniques, the setting in which he works can adversely influence his approach. Thus in a study of general practice (Goldberg and Blackwell, 1970), a general practitioner with considerable psychiatric experience failed to detect a third of the psychiatric morbidity present in his patients. Consideration of the possible reasons for this 'hidden morbidity' suggested that doctors were particularly likely to miss psychological and social problems when the patient presented with somatic symptoms, or when such problems represented an adverse reaction to established physical illness.

This failure to detect important morbidity occurred even when the physical illnesses concerned were known to cause psychological and social problems. Thus, although a considerable proportion of the women who underwent mastectomy for breast cancer developed anxiety, depression, marital and sexual difficulties, it appeared uncommon for surgeons or general practitioners routinely to ask questions designed to elicit the presence or absence of such problems (Maguire, 1975). In consequence the surgeons often remained ignorant of the true impact of the illness on the women and their families. Similarly, direct observation of interviews with women attending a breast clinic for the first time with a breast lump, found that the surgeons inquired directly about the possibility of the women being worried in only 5 per cent of those 69 per cent of cases who were very distressed (Maguire *et al.*, 1975). It also showed that the probability of surgeons attempting to reassure the patient bore no relation to the level of emotional distress reported by the women, and that they often failed to detect or respond to verbal and non-verbal cues. As a result, some of the women were too distressed to provide the relevant information, or register what was said to them about their illnesses and treatments.

While much of the discussion about interviewing difficulties has so far only concerned the detection of psychological and social problems, it should be stressed that problems relating to physical illness were also likely to be missed. Such omission appeared most probable when the patients clearly had psychiatric difficulties. In a study of 200 consecutive admissions to a psychiatric unit, the physical illness evident in 33 per cent (Maguire and Granville-Grossman, 1968) had only previously been diagnosed in half of these cases. It seemed likely that most doctors tended to assume that clinical problems would fall into either a physical or psychological domain and would only rarely utilize an interviewing strategy that allowed for the possibility of both types of problem being present.

This apparent tendency of doctors to direct their questions to one kind of problem or the other, appeared to be paralleled by patients' attitudes. Even when the surgeons in the breast clinic study did ask patients how they were feeling in an attempt to assess their mental state, the patients invariably replied in terms of their physical health. When asked about this they gave three reasons. They considered that the surgeons' main concerns were with their physical health, that they had no right to burden the surgeons with their worries, and there was probably little that could be done to alleviate their distress. This pessimism about the possibility of effective treatments was also given as a principal reason why patients in the twelve months before their deaths failed to report distressing physical and psychiatric symptoms to their general practitioners (Cartwright *et al.*, 1973).

These findings strongly suggested that doctors ought to be trained to adopt a more holistic interviewing approach and to educate their patients to realize that they were genuinely concerned with practical, social, and psychological problems as well as physical illness.

Inadequacies of traditional methods of interview training

This review coupled with further discussions with medical students suggested that there were three main reasons for this lack of basic interviewing skills in medical students and doctors.

The lack of time and priority given to interview training

Despite the obvious relevance of interviewing skills to clinical practice, few medical schools devoted much curriculum time to interview training. Where courses in interviewing were held they were usually very short, given at the outset of the students' clinical course, and took the form of a few formal lectures and demonstrations. They placed the emphasis on teaching students the repertoires of questions that should be asked about a patient's physical health and on how to carry out a clinical examination. Little attention was generally paid to teaching students how they should actually conduct their interviews. Few students received any further interview training, after these introductory courses. Their teachers appeared to assume that the students would develop their interviewing skills automatically as a consequence of their other clinical training.

The lack of an appropriate interviewing model

A further problem concerned the conflicting advice medical students were given about what questions to ask and how to interview. While the questions to be asked of physically ill patients were usually made explicit and covered repeatedly, they received much less guidance about obtaining social and personal histories. Indeed, the handouts they received often contained scant reference to these more personal matters. Thus, the interviewing model they initially learned was heavily 'organic' in its orientation. In consequence the students felt that they should not routinely pay more than lip-service to the psychological and social aspects of a case, particularly as they were also sometimes actively discouraged by their tutors from asking questions about these areas. When they began their psychiatric clerkship they found exactly the opposite emphasis, their tutors arguing the importance of routine inquiry about a patient's mental state, psychological and social adjustment. Hence when they returned to the general medical and surgical wards they found themselves in considerable conflict over what questions to ask, particularly as they had difficulty integrating the two approaches. Where students did succeed in evolving a method that allowed them to cover organic, social, and psychological matters, they usually discovered that the psychological and social data that they reported back went unheeded by their teachers. Inevitably this caused them to question the relevance and appropriateness of a psychological and social approach in the general hospital setting. It also reactivated worries that such an approach may after all be 'traumatic' to the patient, despite their contrary experience during the psychiatric clerkship. As a result the students tended to adopt either an 'organic' approach or a 'psychiatric' one, according to the setting in which they worked and the type of patient they thought they were dealing with. Unfortunately, this dichotomous approach was often inappropriate to their patients' real needs. They urgently needed a more appropriate interviewing model.

Lack of direct observation and feedback

The students' uncertainty about how to interview was heightened by the absence of any feedback from their teachers about their interview performances. Such feedback was rare because few teachers ever observed their students carrying out an interview. Instead they assessed their students' skills on the basis of what they reported back to them about the histories they obtained. Yet it had been reported that judgements made on this basis correlated poorly with students' actual interview behaviour (Muslin *et al.*, 1968). Thus it was quite possible for a student who was poor at relating to his patients to give a good performance on a ward round and seriously mislead his teachers as to his interviewing abilities (Hinz, 1966). Hence students gained little idea of how they actually appeared to their patients. Any bad habits they had developed, such as neglecting to introduce themselves or not giving their patients sufficient time to answer their questions remained undetected.

Development of an interviewing model

In view of these deficiencies it was considered that the first priority was to develop an interviewing model which would provide medical students with explicit guidelines about the way they should obtain a history of the present illness. It was agreed that the model should take account of the particular interviewing skills that seemed to be lacking in medical students and doctors, be geared to the time they would have for their interviews after qualification, be flexible enough to allow for the range and complexity of the clinical problems they would encounter and heed previous accounts of interviewing procedures (Morgan and Engel, 1969; Goldberg and Blackwell, 1970). Early experience of using this model suggested that students were helped by the inclusion of examples of particular pitfalls, and assimilated it more easily when it was presented in two distinct parts, the data that should be obtained and the interviewing techniques that should be used.

The data that should be obtained

Details of the main problems

NATURE OF THE CURRENT PROBLEMS. The first task of the interviewer is to help the patient communicate the nature of his current problems and to ensure that these are properly clarified before he pursues any other material. He should be particularly aware of the possibility that the patient may have several problems, that these may be physical, social, or psychological in nature, and that patients sometimes initially volunteer a problem that masks the difficulties they really wish to communicate to the doctor. After the patient has mentioned his problems the interviewer should ask whether there are any other problems the patient has been experiencing and would like to mention. This minimizes the risk that important problems will remain undisclosed.

Once he feels he has a grasp of the nature and range of the patient's problems, the interviewer should summarize them in a way which includes a further check on the existence of other problems. For example, 'you mentioned that you have been troubled by chest pain and breathlessness for the last month. Has there been anything else that has been bothering you that you have not yet mentioned?'

By this stage the interviewer should be in a position to decide which of the problems he can deal with within the time he has available. It should be noted that patients may on some occasions present with a perfectly straightforward complaint, for example, an attack of 'flu' or earache due to otitis media. In these circumstances the interviewer may not feel it appropriate to probe for the existence of other problems. However, if he is in any doubt he should err on the side of assuming there may be other problems.

The interviewer should then try to establish, for each problem elicited, the following information:

THE TIME OF ONSET. The interviewer should take care to obtain the exact dates when each of the main problems started. Patients can often date what has happened recently very accurately providing the interviewer encourages them to do so and does not too easily accept that they cannot remember.

THE SUBSEQUENT DEVELOPMENT OF THE PROBLEMS. When clear onsets have been established the interviewer should find out how the problems have developed over the period between onset and the time of interview. He should be on the look-out for evidence of any change points, that is any occasion when there was any major change in the intensity and frequency of the problem. For these may provide important aetiological clues.

PRECIPITATING OR RELIEVING FACTORS. The interviewer should next inquire whether the patient feels that the onset or major changes in his particular problems were related to any particular factors. Where factors are volunteered, for example 'overwork' the interviewer should clarify just what changes occurred at work prior to the onset of the problem. He must be concerned to guard against the tendency of people to account for problems by blaming recent events, even though these events bear no real relationship to the problems. He can best do this by dating the timing of onsets and alleged 'causal' factors carefully.

For example, in one interview a patient volunteered that his attacks of chest pain were definitely caused by his having started a new and more physically demanding job. Since this claim seemed very plausible, the interviewer accepted it at face value. However, had he checked the dates of starting the job and the onset of chest pains he would have found the chest pains preceded the new job by some six months. Had he also inquired whether there was anything else associated with the attacks of pain he would have discovered that they were related to times when the patient was reminded of his wife's death. She had died a year previously of a coronary. This patient turned out not to have any organic disease, and his complaints were found to stem from an unresolved grief reaction and subsequent depressive illness.

THE HELP GIVEN TO DATE. Once the roles of any possible contributory factors have been identified correctly, the interviewer should ask whether the patient has already been given any help with his problems. Where help has been given the interviewer must try to establish the exact nature, dose, duration, clinical, and unwanted effects of each episode of treatment given. This will help him avoid prescribing a course of treatment which has not worked before. It may also suggest better methods of approach. The interviewer should realize that even if patients cannot recall the exact name of the pills they are on, they can often describe the pills and the frequency with which they take them. They may even have the appropriate medication with them at the interview.

AVAILABILITY OF SUPPORT. The degree of practical and emotional support available to a patient may determine how he copes with his problems and whether he requires hospital admission or not. The interviewer should, therefore, ask the patient whether he has anyone he feels he can discuss his problems with and who he usually turns to for advice. He should be particularly concerned to establish whether close relatives, especially spouses, have been supportive to the patient in his attempts to cope with his current problems.

The impact of the problems on the patient and the family. Many types of problem, particularly established physical and psychiatric illnesses may have an adverse effect on the day-to-day functioning of the patient and other family members. Since these effects may be quite serious, cause considerable family problems, and yet remain undisclosed by the patient, the possibility of their existence must be inquired about. The interviewer should inquire whether the problems have had any adverse effects on the following areas: the patient's ability to do his job, and his level of job satisfaction; his ability to cope with his day-to-day chores; his ability to pursue and enjoy his usual hobbies, leisure and social activities; the quality of his relationships with his wife, immediate family, and other close relatives, as judged by his usual feelings for these people, the frequency of his contacts with them, experience of any rows or friction; his interest in, enjoyment of, and frequency of sexual relations; and his mood, that is, the way he has been feeling in his spirits.

Where any mood change has occurred to an extent greater than can be accounted for by the normal variation in the patient's mood, its nature and extent must be properly clarified by the interviewer.

When the predominant mood change is one of depression the interviewer should screen for the possibility of other depressive symptoms, particularly loss of appetite, weight, sleep disturbance, diurnal variation, change in bowel habits, loss of energy, and suicidal ideas. When suicidal ideas are admitted, the interviewer must ask questions that allow him to assess the risk of suicide. These should include inquiry about previous suicide attempts, the presence of ideas of hopelessness, worthlessness, guilt, being a burden, and fears of bodily illness. The assessment of suicidal risk in anyone who reports depression is stressed because of its importance and because it is thought that many suicides could be prevented if doctors made such routine inquiry of depressed patients.

At the completion of this phase of the interview the interviewer should have obtained as vivid and reliable a picture of what life has been like for the patient and his family since the onset of the main problems. This will allow the interviewer to determine what needs to be done to resolve any difficulties caused by these problems.

The patient's view of his problems. The interviewer should next try to find out what ideas and attitudes the patient has about the nature and likely outcome of his problems. For only by obtaining a clear understanding of these can the interviewer hope to provide effective reassurance and remove any misconceptions that could be a bar to recovery or to compliance with advice and treatment.

For example, a patient who presented with complaints of severe headaches was privately terrified that he might have a brain tumour, since his father had died from cancer. He was not reassured by a flat statement from the doctor that there was nothing to worry about. However, had the doctor concerned taken care to find out first how anxious the patient was and why, he would have recognized the need to explain carefully why he knew it was not due to a tumour.

Another example concerned a patient who had been admitted to hospital with a myocardial infarction. He had been led to believe by a nurse that it was of a minor nature. He was, therefore, unwilling to comply with the advice that he should restrict his physical activities considerably. The doctor who next interviewed him failed to realize this patient's attitude to his illness and reasons for it. He wrongly interpreted the patient's lack of compliance as just bloody-mindedness.

Predisposition to develop similar problems. In order to put the problems, their effects, and the patient's attitudes into perspective, the interviewer should next try to learn whether such problems and reactions could have been predicted from a knowledge of the kind of person the patient was before the onset of the current difficulties. In particular he should determine whether the patient and his close relatives have had similar problems before, whether these were triggered by similar events and had the same consequences. The interviewer should also obtain some idea of the patient's personality before the onset of the problems. The extent to which he does this will be governed by whether he has any prior knowledge of the patient and the nature of the problems the patient is complaining of. Where the interviewer elicits a psychological problem or wants to predict how the patient may cope with his problem he should elicit the following data: details of his family of origin, their occupation, attitudes to the patient, physical and psychological health; the patient's early development and childhood; schooling, further education, sexual development, job history, interpersonal relationships including marriage, leisure interests, social activities; previous health and characteristic reactions to particular types of stress.

Screening questions. The full range of the patient's problem should now be clear. It is, however, possible that some patients may still not have felt able to communicate one or more key problems. The interviewer needs some way of routinely screening for this possibility.

If the focus in an interview has been on physical problems and the patient has denied that the physical problems have affected his mood, the interviewer should, if still in any doubt, ask whether the patient has noticed any change in the way he has been feeling in his spirits.

Similarly if psychological or social problems have been emphasized questions should be asked about the patient's physical well-being, and if necessary a systematic review of the main physical systems carried out. Where appropriate the interviewer may wish to carry out a more thorough review of his patient's mental state. Details of this can be found in the relevant psychiatric textbooks.

The interviewing techniques that should be used

The interviewer will find it helpful to divide his interview into four parts, the beginning, explaining the purpose of the interview and the procedure to be followed, obtaining the relevant information, and terminating the interview.

Beginning the interview. In view of the evidence that this part of the interview is often neglected by both medical students and clinicians, it is suggested that the interviewer should take particular care to:

GREET THE PATIENT. The interviewer should stand up as the patient enters the consulting room, move toward the patient, greet him verbally; with a clear 'Hello' or 'Good morning', using his correct name and title, and shake hands.

SEATING THE PATIENT. Once the greeting is completed the interviewer should indicate clearly by words and gesture where the patient is to sit. He should then sit down himself, adopting a body posture that conveys an attitude of interest and friendliness to the patient, for example by leaning slightly forward in his chair, looking directly at the patient and smiling. He should try to avoid extreme postures such as lounging back in the chair in a very casual manner, or leaning so far forward that the patient feels uneasy or intimidated.

SELF-INTRODUCTION. Once the patient and interviewer are comfortably seated the latter should introduce himself by name and explain exactly what his status is. For example he might say, 'I am Dr Smith,

Mr Morris's registrar' or 'I am Tom Brown, a medical student working with Dr Jones'. He should avoid the temptation of trying to introduce himself while he and the patient are still in the process of sitting down. Otherwise it is unlikely that the patient will register what he says.

Discussing the purpose of the interview and the procedure to be followed. (*Note*. We consider it useful to spend some time explaining to the patient the kinds of information we need to know if we are going to be able to help them. For we believe that patients will be more co-operative and more likely to produce the necessary data if we do so. We also consider that patients benefit from knowing the time that is available for their interviews. For they can then pace their contributions more effectively, indicate that the time offered is insufficient for their needs, or suggest it is far more than necessary.) Thus the interviewer should next:

(i) Explain the exact purpose of his interview. For example, 'I would like to find out as much as possible about your present problems, in the time we have available'.

(ii) Mention the time that is available if needed. Thus the interviewer might say 'we have about fifteen minutes to do this if we need it'.

(iii) Add that he needs to make a few notes to help him remember details of what is discussed and that these will be confidential.

(iv) Inquire whether what he proposes to do is acceptable to the patient and meets his requirements. He should do this in a manner that encourages the patient to realize that the interviewer is genuinely interested in his viewpoint. Having made this inquiry he must also give the patient time to reply. For only in this way can he adapt his approach to the patient's real needs. It may well be that the patient will indicate that certain aspects of the procedure are unacceptable. For example, a patient may object to the note-taking. The interviewer can then make allowance for this, or go into the patient's objection more deeply in an effort to change his mind. He should thus prevent the patient being very inhibited by the note-taking.

(v) Finally, the interviewer should ensure that the patient is as much at ease as possible before he continues the interview. He should be on the look-out for any sign that the patient is uneasy about the situation in which the interview is being carried out. For example, he may note that the patient keeps glancing at the telephone which has already rung once, but been left unanswered. When he asks if the patient feels able to carry on with the interview he is not surprised that the patient says he is afraid of repeated interruptions. He can then ask that no calls be put through for the next ten minutes.

(*Note*. So far the advice given has been based on the assumption that the interview will be carried out in a consulting room. However, many interviews have to be conducted at the patient's bedside and some minor changes in the procedure are necessary. The interviewer should obviously take the initiative in approaching and greeting the patient, and adopting an appropriate sitting position so that the patient can see him without difficulty. He should pay particular attention to the patient's attitude to being interviewed in such a public situation. For it is common for patients to be reluctant to talk about personal matters if they know they can be overheard by patients in the beds on either side of them. Thus, given the chance to say how they feel about the interview situation they may ask the interviewer to draw the curtains round or to find somewhere more private.)

Obtaining the relevant information. In this, the main part of the interview, the interviewer should begin by using a question which will encourage the patient to outline his key problems. Thus the interviewer may ask 'can you begin by telling me what problems brought you to the hospital', or ' . . . to see me'. He should then ask 'has anything else been worrying or bothering you?' By this stage of the interview he should have some feel of the personality of the patient he is dealing with and be in a position to decide what interviewing approach might be effective. For example, if the patient is being very pedantic and keeps going into excessive detail, the interviewer may decide to explain that he does not need the patient to be so detailed in his answers. Alternatively, if the patient takes a long time to answer, the fact that he has already agreed to some time limit can be used to try to encourage him to speed up his replies.

Whatever the difficulties posed by individual patients the interviewer should try to encourage the patient to give his story in his own words, as vividly but accurately as possible. He should do so by:

FACILITATION. Facilitation takes two forms: verbal and non-verbal.

Verbal. This concerns encouraging the patient to continue talking about relevant matters by saying 'go on', 'can you tell me more about that?', 'what happened then', or 'You mentioned that you felt a pain in your chest'. It requires the interviewer to keep silent after making such a prompt, so that the patient will continue his story. There is a strong tendency for many interviewers to jump in too soon after making such a facilitating comment.

Non-verbal. The interviewer may also facilitate by nodding his head and looking attentive. This applies particularly when the patient comes to the end of a statement. For at that point he is likely to look up for signs of approval or disapproval of what he has said.

LISTENING. The interviewer should allow the patient to talk without unnecessary and inappropriate interruptions, providing of course that what is being said is relevant. He should avoid the tendency of many interviewers to ask a further question before the patient has had a chance to reply. He should not be afraid of pauses or silences and indeed may find them useful to give himself time to assimilate what has been said, or think about where he has got to in the interview.

ENCOURAGING THE PATIENT TO BE RELEVANT BY: Being alert to occasions when the patient gets off the point. Taking action to bring the patient back to the point by interruption and redirection, for example, 'What you say is interesting, but it would be helpful at this point if we could return to what you were saying about your chest pain—we can deal with your . . . later.' Reclarifying the nature of information you want from the patient. 'I wonder if I could just explain again what it would help me to know about your . . .'

HELPING THE PATIENT TO DESCRIBE THE REAL NATURE, DEVELOPMENT, AND QUALITY OF HIS PROBLEMS BY: Asking the patient to provide actual examples of the problems and their effect, for example, 'when you say you were sleeping badly over the last week, can you describe a typical night from the time you went to bed until 8 am in the morning?' or 'When you say attacks of pain, can you describe just what they are like?'

AVOIDING JARGON. It is all too easy for the interviewer and patient to believe they share assumptions about the meanings of words and to fail to realize there may be wide differences between them in their interpretation of particular terms. The interviewer should, therefore, avoid the use of jargon and should not accept any words used by the patient he does not fully understand. For example, one patient volunteered 'I have had the most terrible diarrhoea'. The interviewer assumed she meant looseness and frequency of bowel habits. In fact had he clarified what she meant he would have discovered that she meant she'd been very irregular, and passing pus and blood in her stools.

PAYING ATTENTION TO IMPORTANT LEADS. In the course of an interview patients will give several hints by the words they use or changes in voice, facial expression, posture, about other problems or their feelings about current difficulties. The interviewer should be alert to these and try to pursue them. In general he will be inclined to avoid doing so and in consequence will miss important information. For example, when a woman complained of abdominal pain and was asked if anyone in her family had had similar trouble, she mentioned that her father had died of cancer of the stomach ten months ago. As she did so she became very distressed and tearful. She then made a very obvious effort to pull herself together. The interviewer decided not to comment on her distress because he wanted to avoid her becoming more upset. He went on to interview her in a way that concentrated solely on the possible physical diagnoses. Yet had he said 'you seemed upset when you talked of your father', she would have responded by saying she had not been able to get over his death, that previous tests have found nothing wrong physically, and that her pains were identical to those suffered by her father. This would have led him to consider the correct diagnosis of atypical grief.

AVOID USING AN UNSATISFACTORY QUESTION STYLE. The interviewer should avoid putting questions in a form that presupposes an answer or restricts the information given. Thus he should ask 'how have your water-works been' rather than 'You have been passing water frequently?' He should also avoid asking questions which force the patient to choose between unsuitable alternatives, for example, 'was it because you walked too quickly or ate too much' when both of these had precipitated the pain involved.

It is also important to put questions one at a time so that each point is answered rather than to bombard the patient with several questions at once, for example, 'were you losing weight, or appetite and did you have any cough'. For if multiple questions are used there is a risk that only one element in the question will be responded to and the interviewer will fail to realize that the others have not been answered satisfactorily.

AVOID CONFUSION IN THE STORY OBTAINED. The interviewer should explain to the patient right at the start that he should try to be precise about the information he gives, especially the dating of key symptoms, problems, stressful events, and the nature of any previous treatments. He will find that in attempting to establish the relation between problems and stressful events, the use of certain anchor dates (for example holidays and birthdays) will be helpful. He should also be particularly alert to any uncertainties that arise in the interview. For example, 'I'm not clear what you meant by that, could you explain it again' or 'I'm still a bit confused about when your problems started. Could we try and get that clear before we go any further.'

Terminating the interview. The interviewer should leave sufficient time for him to end his interview properly within the agreed time-limits. Two to three minutes will usually be enough. He should explain to the patient that he would like to go over the story so far obtained in order to check its accuracy and correct any gross distortions. He should then ask whether anything important has been missed out and whether the patient would like to ask anything of him. He should then end the interview on time, with a clear concluding statement, and avoid being drawn into any further conversations by the patient.

Development and evaluation of an interview training procedure

In view of this lack of any systematic opportunity for students to practise their interviewing techniques and the neglect of direct observation and feedback, it was considered that the training procedure should include the following components: a practice interview with a real patient under a strict time-limit where the goal was to obtain a precise and relevant history of the patient's current problems; presentation of the interviewing model in the form of a printed handout; and videotape feedback and discussion of the interview performance with the student. Videotape replay was chosen as the mode of feedback because its use allowed attention to be paid both to verbal and non-verbal behaviours and appeared acceptable to medical students (Suess, 1970).

Preliminary experiences in using this procedure with medical students during their psychiatric clerkship suggested that it was very much appreciated by them and led to an improvement in their interviewing skills. However, since students were taught on an individual basis the training procedure was time-consuming. Hence it was felt that its continued use could only be justified if it proved superior to traditional methods. An experiment was therefore carried out to compare the effects of the procedure on students' interviewing skills with those due to traditional training alone.

Twenty-four clinical students were allocated randomly to an experimental or control group. Both groups had already received interview training based on what they reported back from their contacts with patients and participated in a few seminars on medical and psychiatric history-taking. They could thus be said to have experienced the usual training given in interviewing.

Each student in the experimental group was first asked to interview a different psychiatric patient for fifteen minutes in order to obtain a history of the present illness. They were informed that their interviews would be recorded on videotape for later playback and that they should write up a careful history afterwards. Immediately after this interview, each student was given a handout describing the interviewing model, and then shown his interview on television. He was asked to consider the problems it revealed and to compare what he did with the suggested model.

Students in the traditional group were given an identical interview task but told that their feedback and presentation of the model would be delayed until they had completed a second interview. The patients given to them were matched with those given to the experimental group for degree of difficulty.

A week later each of the students in the two groups carried out a similar test interview, but with a different patient from the one they had previously seen. Their performances were judged on the basis of the amount of accurate and relevant information contained in the case-histories, and on ratings made by the patients. The main finding was that the experimental group obtained three times as much relevant and accurate information as the control students, a difference which was very significant ($p < 0.001$). It was also evident that this improvement had not been gained at the expense of the patients' feelings. For the experimental group tended to obtain more favourable patient ratings than the control group.

While these findings confirmed the effectiveness of the training procedure it was not clear how much each component contributed to this. A second experiment was therefore carried out to compare the effects of presentation of the model with those due to the model plus feedback (Rutter and Maguire, 1975). While this showed that both the presentation of an explicit model and feedback of performance played an important part in the gain in interviewing skills, the model coupled with the opportunity to practise under strictly controlled conditions made the major contribution.

It thus seemed useful to consider how the modelling component might be made more effective, especially since it relied only on the presentation and discussion of a printed handout. It was thought that students would benefit from watching teachers using the interviewing model with real patients (Enelow *et al.*, 1970). Appropriate demonstration videotapes were therefore made.

Another issue concerned the timing of the interview training. The students on the psychiatric clerkship repeatedly commented that it should be given at the outset of their clinical training when they most needed guidance and before they had developed any bad interviewing habits. It was, therefore, decided to use these tapes during an introductory course on psychological aspects of medicine and to evaluate their use (Maguire *et al.*, 1975).

Thirty medical students were randomly allocated either to a control group or to one of two experimental groups. After a pre-course assessment of their interviewing skills using the same methods as in the previous experiments, the control group attended three seminars on psychological aspects of medicine and interviewing techniques. These seminars followed a similar pattern to previous courses. Training was based on observation and discussion of interviews conducted by the teacher or students with psychiatric patients in front of the group. The control group were not presented with the interviewing model, although the teacher was given identical interviewing objectives to those followed by the teacher of the experimental groups.

The experimental groups had two teaching sessions. The first session concerned the presentation and discussion of videotapes and a handout describing the topics that should be covered in a history of present illness. This was followed by a test-interview where each student was asked to interview one of two simulated patients who were programmed to reproduce identical cases, in order to practise covering the essential topics. The second teaching session focused on the presentation and discussion of tapes depicting how the interview should be conducted.

After these courses were completed, both control and experimental groups conducted a second test-interview with one of a different pair of simulated patients. Their performances in these interviews were judged on the following criteria: the amount of accurate and relevant information obtained, ratings made by the simulated patients, and independent ratings of the videotapes.

It was found that the experimental groups performed significantly better than the control group on all the three outcome measures. By contrast to the control group, the experimental groups showed a significant improvement both in the amount of information they obtained and the behaviours which they used between their first and second test-interviews.

It thus appeared that the use of videotape recordings to demonstrate an interview model, coupled with an opportunity to practise under strictly controlled conditions, was much superior to a traditional seminar approach in helping medical students develop basic interviewing skills. The experiment also demonstrated that the model could be effectively presented on a group basis and that the use of simulated patients was both feasible and acceptable.

Future developments

A major problem to be faced is how a training procedure such as the one outlined here can be adapted for use with large numbers of medical students. It was therefore encouraging to find that an interview rating scale developed to measure interviewing skills could be used reliably by non-medically trained people. For this suggests that students could learn to rate their own performances. This finding coupled with the successful use of simulated patients raises the possibility that an independent learning programme could be established which would consist of videotaped presentation of an interviewing model on a group basis, individual practice with simulated patients, followed by feedback and self-rating.

Before such a programme can be mounted, three main issues require clarification. First, it needs to be determined what the mode of feedback of performance should be. For it could be that videotape feedback is not very much better than audio feedback, or direct comment by an instructor at this basic level of interviewing skills. Second, while the use of simulators result in a gain in skills it is not yet clear how much such skills generalize to work with real patients. Third, it remains to be seen how well students can rate themselves or each other's interviews.

Whatever the answers to these questions turn out to be, it does seem that the provision of a clear interviewing model, opportunity to practise interviewing skills under strictly controlled conditions, feedback and discussion of performance do lead to a striking improvement in the level of medical students' interviewing skills.

Acknowledgements

The work described in this paper was carried out in the Department of Psychiatry, University of Oxford. We are particularly grateful to Professor Michael Gelder for his guidance and encouragement, Mr Charles Engel, Dr Don Clarke, and Mr Brian Jolley of BMA/British Life Assurance Trust Centre for Educational Development for their collaboration in the simulator experiment, Mr Paul Skinner for his technical help and all the medical students who acted as 'guinea-pigs' in these experiments.

References

ANDERSON, J., DAY, J. L., DOWLING, M. A. C., and PETTINGALE, K. W. (1970). 'The definition and evaluation of the skills required to obtain a patient's history of illness: the use of videotape recordings', *Postgrad. med. J.* **46**, 606–12.

CARTWRIGHT, A., HOCKEY, L., and ANDERSON, J. L. (1973). *Life before Death* (London: Routledge and Kegan Paul).

ENELOW, A. J., ADLER, L. M., and WEXLER, M. (1970). 'Programmed instruction in interviewing', *J. Am. med. Ass.* **212**, 1843–6.

GOLDBERG, D. P., and BLACKWELL, B. (1970). 'Psychiatric illness in general practice: a detailed study using a new method of case identification', *Br. med. J.* **2**, 439–41.

HELFER, R. E. (1970). 'An objective comparison of the paediatric interviewing skills of freshmen and senior medical students', *Paediatrics*, **45**, 623–7.

HINZ, C. F. (1966). 'Direct observation as a means of teaching and evaluating clinical skills', *J. med. Educ.* **41**, 150–61.

KORSCH, B. M., GOZZI, E. K., and FRANCIS, V. (1968). 'Gaps in doctor–patient communications. I. Doctor–patient interaction and patient satisfaction', *Paediatrics*, **42**, 855–71.

74   *Training medical students to communicate*

MacNamara, M. (1974). 'Talking with patients: some problems met by medical students', *Br. J. med. Educ.* **8**, 17–23.

Maguire, G. P. (1975). 'Psychological and social consequences of breast cancer', *Nursing Mirror*, 3 April.

—— and Granville-Grossman, K. L. (1968). 'Physical illness in psychiatric patients', *Br. J. Psychiat.* **114**, 1365–9.

—— Julier, D. L., Hawton, K. E., and Bancroft, J. H. J. (1974). 'Psychiatric morbidity and referral on two general medical wards', *Br. med. J.* **1**, 268–70.

—— Clarke, D., and Jolly, B. (1975). 'An experimental comparison of three methods of presenting an interview procedure to beginning medical students' (to be published).

—— Lee, E., Bevington, D., Cornell, C., and Kuchemann, C. (1975). 'Emotional distress and communications within a breast clinic' (to be published).

Morgan, W. L., and Engel, G. L. (1969). *Clinical Approach to the Patient* (Philadelphia: W. D. Saunders).

Muslin, H. L., Singer, P. R., Meuser, M. F., and Leahy, J. P. (1968). 'Research and learning in psychiatric interviewing', *J. med. Educ.* **43**, 398–403.

Rutter, D. R., and Maguire, G. P. (1975). 'The experimental evaluation of a method of interview training for medical students' (to be published).

Suess, J. F. (1970). 'Self-confrontation of videotaped psychotherapy as a teaching device for psychiatric students', *J. med. Educ.* **45**, 271–82.

Tapia, F. (1972). 'Teaching medical interviewing: a practical technique', *Br. J. med. Educ.* **6**, 133–6.

Towards better doctor–patient communications

Contributions from social and experimental psychology

Philip Ley
Senior Lecturer in Clinical Psychology
Sub-Department of Clinical Psychology
University of Liverpool

Towards better doctor–patient communications

The problems

From Fletcher's (1973) review of communication in medicine it is clear that the field of doctor–patient communication is a very wide one which is amenable to study by many different methods. The investigations to be described are limited to two main problems. The first of these is the problem of patients' dissatisfaction with the communication aspect of their hospital stay, and the second the problem of patients not following advice given to them.

A summary of evidence on patients' dissatisfaction with communications has been provided by Ley (1972a). Some of this evidence is summarized in Table 1 below.

It can be seen that substantial numbers of patients are dissatisfied with the communications aspect of their hospital stay. Investigations by Carstairs (1970) and Raphael (1967) using different methodologies, which do not permit one to assess the percentage of patients dissatisfied, also provide evidence of patients' frequent dissatisfaction with communications. Finally the survey commissioned by the Committee

Table 1. *Surveys of satisfaction with communications*

Investigator	Length of time between discharge and follow-up	Possible respondents replying %	Dissatisfied %
McGhee (1961)	10–14 days	100	65
Hugh Jones *et al.* (1964)	4 weeks	99	39
Cartwright (1964)	Up to 6 months	70	29
Spelman *et al.* (1965)	Up to 4 weeks	100	54
Houghton (1968)	3–8 weeks	92	35*
Raphael (1969)	Immediately before or after discharge	62	18
United Manchester Hospitals (1970)	2–5 days	50	11*

* These studies reported several satisfaction rates so their median figures are given here.

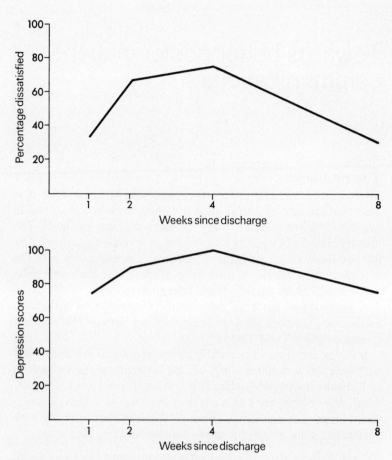

Fig. 1. *Dissatisfaction with communications and depression in relation to time since discharge from hospital*

on Hospital Complaints Procedure and reported by the Department of Health and Social Security (1973) found that 22 per cent of in-patients felt that they had been inadequately informed about their illness, and 18 per cent about their treatment. Inspection of the data in Table 1 reveals three possible trends. There appears to be a drop in dissatisfaction over the period 1961–70. Secondly, there appears to be an inverse relationship between proportion of patients replying and dissatisfaction rates. Thirdly, there appears to be a curvilinear relationship between time since discharge from hospital and reported dissatisfaction. These are all confounded with one another in the summarized data. Ley *et al.* (1976) provide evidence to show that only the third of these apparent trends is real. Fig. 1 shows the proportions of medical in-patients reporting satisfaction with communications after various lengths of time since discharge from hospital.

These temporal changes in satisfaction appear to be associated with mood changes following discharge. Patients come out of hospital feeling in reasonably good spirits and then become more depressed for a period before returning to normal mood. Mood changes as measured by the Hildreth Feeling Scale (Hildreth, 1946), are also shown in Fig. 1.

The existence of patients' dissatisfaction with communication could, of course, be a problem with a simple solution. The usual reasons advanced to explain dissatisfaction have been listed by Ley and Spelman (1967) as shortage of time; the belief that patients do not want to know; patients' diffidence; errors; reactionary attitudes; and organizational factors. If these reasons were adequate explanations the solution to the problem would be simply for medical and other staff to provide patients with information. However, it is clear that this will not do. The available evidence shows that even when doctors feel that they have made special efforts to inform patients, patients remain dissatisfied (Hugh Jones *et al.*, 1964; Spelman *et al.*, 1966) and even when explicit action is taken to improve communications patients remain dissatisfied (Houghton, 1968). To reinforce this point Table 2 provides a rearrangement of the studies mentioned earlier, to show the lack of effect of simple efforts to inform the patient.

Table 2. *The effects of special efforts to inform patients on dissatisfaction with communications*

	Dissatisfied %
Studies reporting no special efforts	
McGhee (1961)	65
Cartwright (1964)	29
Raphael (1969)	18
United Manchester Hospitals (1970)	5–17
Department of Health and Social Security (1973)	18–22
Studies reporting special efforts	
Hugh Jones *et al.* (1964)	39
Spelman *et al.* (1966)	54
Houghton (1968)	35

Table 3. *The frequency with which patients fail to follow medical advice*

Type of advice	No. of studies	Patients who did not follow the advice %		
		Range	*Mean*	*Median*
Medicine-taking				
1. PAS and other TB drugs	20	8–76	37·5	35·0
2. Antibiotics	8	11–92	48·7	50·0
3. Psychiatric drugs	9	11–51	38·6	44·0
4. Other medicines, eg antacids, iron	12	9–87	47·7	57·5
Diet	11	20–84	49·4	45·0
Other advice, eg child care, antenatal exercises	8	30–79	54·6	51·0
All advice	68	8–92	44·0	44·3

The second problem is that of patients' non-compliance with advice given to them. A tabular summary of published studies up to the end of 1970 is given by Ley (1972*b*). This is reproduced in Table 3.

This evidence shows that a very large proportion of patients will not follow advice given to them.

The causes

Reasons for patients' dissatisfaction with communications and failure to follow advice

Four main theories have been put forward to explain the failures of communication implied by patients' dissatisfaction and patients' non-compliance.

The first of these can be labelled the 'personality hypothesis'. This states that patients who are dissatisfied with communications or who fail to follow advice will differ in personality and/or attitude and/or demographic characteristics from those who are satisfied and those who do follow advice. For example, Davis (1968*a*) states: 'It is hypothesized that selected patient characteristics will explain variations in behavioural and attitudinal compliance.'

Table 4. *Comparisons of scores of satisfied and dissatisfied patients on Cattell's Sixteen Personality Factor Questionnaire*

Factor	Satisfied patients Mean	SD	Dissatisfied patients Mean	SD
A. Warm, outgoing	5·67	2·43	6·18	2·28
B. Intelligent	5·36	2·11	5·56	1·91
C. Emotionally mature	3·64	1·80	4·41	2·41
E. Self-assured	6·22	1·81	6·22	2·01
F. Not depressed	4·00	2·04	4·67	2·48
G. Conscientious	6·22	1·81	6·70	2·12
H. Adventurous	4·47	1·69	4·78	2·13
I. Dependent	6·44	1·71	6·96	2·01
L. Irritable	6·39	1·62	6·63	1·85
M. Unconventional	5·19	1·91	5·26	2·01
N. Exact, ambitious	6·11	1·91	6·11	1·81
O. Worrying, anxious	6·75	2·15	7·41	1·91
Q1. Experimenting	5·50	1·99	5·33	2·42
Q2. Self-sufficient	5·03	2·52	4·74	2·95
Q3. Controlled	4·39	1·90	4·96	2·08
Q4. Tense	6·92	2·13	8·07	1·68
Anxiety	7·42	1·71	7·59	1·91
Extraversion	4·56	1·95	5·11	2·17

This possibility has been investigated in our studies of patients' satisfaction with communications. Table 4 shows the mean scores of satisfied and dissatisfied patients on the personality variables measured by Cattell's Sixteen Personality Factor Questionnaire, which is probably the most comprehensive objective measure of personality traits available (Cattell, 1973). It can be seen that the personality scores of satisfied and dissatisfied patients are almost identical. However it was found that satisfied patients were significantly older than dissatisfied ones (Ley *et al.*, 1974*a*).

Several investigations have found patient characteristics to be related to compliance (for example, Davis, 1968*a*; Francis *et al.*, 1969), and in our investigations it has been found that Rotter's Internal–External control variable has been significantly related to compliance in obese patients (Ley *et al.*, 1976; Tulips *et al.*, 1974).

But even if such relationships are incontrovertibly established knowledge of them is of little practical use. As it is not possible to change such patient characteristics, any relationships found would be limited of value in the control of patients' non-compliance or dissatisfaction.

The remaining three theories are potentially more useful. The first of these is the psychodynamic hypothesis which suggests that the patients presenting complaints is often only a cover for a more deep-seated problem. Communications will fail to the extent that they deal only with the surface problem presented. Whatever the merits of this hypothesis in the general practice situation it seems unlikely that it will apply to many consultations in the hospital situation. It will therefore be considered no further.

The second suggests that patients' dissatisfaction and non-compliance are related to process and interpersonal factors in the communication situation. Very sophisticated research along these lines has been reported by Davis (1968b), Korsch et al. (1968), Francis et al. (1969), and Freemon et al. (1971). These investigators have used Bales's Interaction Process Analysis and factor analytic techniques to specify the dimensions and processes of doctor–patient interaction, and have provided correlational data on the relationship between these variables, satisfaction, and compliance. The hope is that these studies will lead to sufficient understanding for remedial action to be taken where necessary.

The final hypothesis is that of Ley and Spelman (1967) and can be described as the 'cognitive hypothesis'. This states that for 'communication to be effective the message it contains must be understood and remembered, and that many failures in communication are caused by simple failures of comprehension and memory'. These authors did not of course believe that adequate comprehension and memory were sufficient causes for compliance, but argued that they were necessary ones. There are many other variables likely to influence compliance and some of these will be discussed later. The cognitive hypothesis, therefore, directs attention to studies of patients' comprehension and memory.

Patients' understanding of material presented to them

At least three factors are involved in patients' failures to understand. These are that (1) the material presented to patients is often too difficult; (2) patients often lack knowledge; (3) patients are diffident.

The first of these factors has been investigated by examination of

Table 5. *Comprehensibility of some X-ray leaflets as measured by the Flesch Formula*

Leaflet	Population who would be expected to understand it %
Barium meal	75
Barium swallow	75
Bronchogram	40
Cholecystogram	40
Intravenous pyelogram	75

written material prepared for patients. Several techniques are available for assessing the difficulty level of written or spoken material (Ley, 1973). Ley *et al.* (1972) have applied one of these, the Flesch Formula (Flesch, 1948), to some X-ray leaflets issued to patients by a hospital serving a predominantly lower working class area. The Flesch Formula enables one to estimate the percentage of the population who would understand a given piece of writing. Table 5 shows the results of applying this formula to the X-ray leaflets.

These investigators also report the application of the formula to a model barium meal X-ray leaflet proposed by Wild and Evans (1968), which showed that only 24 per cent of the population would be expected to understand it. Similar findings have been reported in studies of leaflets issued by a dental hospital by Lovius *et al.* (1973).

An impressive study of patients' lack of knowledge is that of Boyle (1970). Boyle used a multiple choice technique to assess patients' knowledge of the location of some of their major organs. This technique revealed that many patients thought their organs to be in places other than the correct one.

The percentage of patients wrongly locating the various organs were as follows:

heart	58 per cent	lungs	49 per cent
bladder	40 per cent	intestines	23 per cent
kidneys	54 per cent	liver	51 per cent
stomach	80 per cent	thyroid gland	30 per cent

Unfortunately for the clinician the patients' areas of ignorance lie behind areas of accurate knowledge. Thus, Spelman and Ley (1966) found that amongst a sample of the general population asked questions about lung cancer, 91 per cent knew of the connection with cigarette smoking, 56 per cent knew the symptoms, 73 per cent knew the treatment, but that nearly a third of their sample thought that lung cancer was not very serious and easily curable.

Serious misconceptions on the part of patients were also discovered by Roth *et al.* (1962). In an investigation of patients' beliefs about peptic ulcer it was found that while many patients believed that acid was involved in ulcer formation and maintenance only 10 per cent of the group had a reasonably clear idea that acid was secreted by the stomach. Some patients even thought that acid came from the teeth when they chewed, or their brain when they swallowed. Other examples of patients' lack of knowledge can be found in Ley and Spelman (1967).

The importance of these misunderstandings for the communication process is that they are likely to cause confusion which might well militate against satisfaction and advice. Consider the case of a patient who thinks that (*a*) acid causes ulcers and (*b*) acid is produced by the brain when he swallows. If he is told to eat small, frequent meals, this is in his eyes, tantamount to telling him to put into his stomach frequent doses of what is causing the ulcer. He could, of course, ask questions to dispel his confusion, but it has been widely found that patients are very diffident about asking for information from doctors (Central Health Services Council, 1963; Cartwright, 1964; Ley and Spelman, 1967; Fletcher, 1973). Because patients are diffident the clinician receives no feedback when he produces material which is too difficult, so his performance cannot improve, nor does he have the opportunity to learn what misconceptions his patients have. Indeed, a case could be made out for maintaining that the reduction of patients' diffidence would go a long way to solving the communication problem.

Patients' failure to remember what they are told

A number of studies of patients' failures to remember have been conducted. These are summarized in Table 6.

The number of statements forgotten goes up with the number presented and Ley (1974), provides the following linear regression equation for predicting patients forgetting:

$$Y = 0{\cdot}56X - 0{\cdot}94$$
Where Y = number of statements likely to be forgotten
X = number of statements made to the patient.

Application of this formula to forgetting found in studies reported by Ley and his co-workers shows it to correctly predict the number of statements forgotten plus or minus one with 77 per cent accuracy. In piactice this means that the clinician should expect the patient to forget no statements out of two presented; one out of four presented; two out of six presented, and if eight or more are presented the patient should forget half of what he is told.

Another finding of the investigation of Ley and Spelman (1965), was that advice was more likely to be forgotten than other sorts of statement. Attempts to explain this involved a series of analogue studies in which normal, healthy volunteer subjects were given fictitious medical information to recall. The use of healthy volunteers and fictitious information has great advantages from the point of view of experimental control. It also saves bothering patients with what might turn out to be pointless tasks. The chief danger is that memory for fictitious medical information in volunteers might be quite different from memory for the information amongst patients. This danger has not in fact proved to be a real one. All of the findings of the analogue experiments have been replicable on the real-life situation. Nor are there great differences in amount of forgetting between patients and volunteers. Table 7 provides comparative data on forgetting by volunteers and patients.

The initial analogue studies were designed to test two main

Table 6. *Summary of studies of patients forgetting medical information*

Investigators	Type of patient	Time between consultation and recall	Forgotten %
Ley and Spelman (1965)	47 out-patients	10–80 minutes	37·2
Ley and Spelman (1967)	(a) 22 out-patients	10–80 minutes	38·7
	(b) 22 out-patients	10–80 minutes	40·6
Joyce *et al.* (1969)	(a) 30 out-patients	Immediately after consultation	52·0
	(b) 24 out-patients	1–4 weeks	54·0
Ley *et al.* (1973)	20 general practice patients	Less than 5 minutes	50·0

Table 7. *Forgetting of medical information by volunteers and patients*

Number of statements presented	Number of statements forgotten by	
	Volunteers	Patients
6	2·16	2·42
9	4·23	4·10
12	7·08	5·78

hypotheses: (1) that people recall best what they hear first; (2) that people recall best what they consider most important.

The first of these arose from the observation that the consultant involved in the first investigation of patients' forgetting presented his advice to the patient after he had told the patient the diagnosis and given other information. If there is a primacy effect in recall of medical information the differential forgetting of instructions would be partly explained.

The second hypothesis was a common-sense one. If patients are presented with more material than they can remember, they will start selecting parts of it to remember and discard other parts. The most likely criterion for this selection is the patient's subjective view of the importance of the different statements made to him. He will tend to forget those he thinks unimportant.

To explain the differential forgetting of instructions it was therefore necessary to demonstrate: (1) that laymen consider statements giving advice to be less important than other sorts of medical statement and (2) that there is a correlation between a statement's rated importance and the probability of its recall.

The analogue experiments revealed a strong primacy effect, and the hypothesized relationship between importance and recall (Ley, 1972c). The existence of primacy effects in free recall situations has been known for many years (Jersild, 1929). Recent reviews by Cofer (1972) and Postman (1972) provide summaries of more recent investigations and theoretical explanations.

Some solutions
The control of patients' forgetting

The first attempt to control patients' forgetting arose out of the analogue studies mentioned above. If patients recall best what they are told first and if they remember best what they consider most important, it should be possible to increase recall of instructions and advice either by presenting them first or by stressing their importance. Accordingly three groups of out-patients were compared. The first received the usual procedure, the second had any advice given before other information and the third had advice in its usual place, but with the importance of that advice stressed. The mean percentages of instructions recalled in the three conditions are shown in Table 8.

Table 8. *Recall of advice as a function of method of presentation*

Method of presentation	Recalled %
Normal	44
Advice first	75
Importance of advice stressed	64

However, increased recall of advice was accompanied by decreased recall of other material. It was therefore necessary to find ways of increasing the total amount recalled by patients. Four methods have been tried to date. Three of them stem directly or indirectly from the literature on the experimental psychology of memory and one was discovered serendipitously.

It is well established that meaningful material is more easily remembered than less meaningful material (Jung, 1968). It is also possible to use the Flesch Formula to find easier versions of a piece of writing. The formula as given by Flesch (1948) is:

Reading Ease $= 206 \cdot 84 - 0 \cdot 85W - 1 \cdot 02S$
Where W = average number of syllables per 100 words
S = average length of sentence in words.

The higher the Reading Ease the more easily understood and therefore presumably the more meaningful a piece of writing is. Inspection of the formula shows that to make material easier it is necessary to use shorter words and shorter sentences. A number of experiments have been carried out to assess the effects on total amount remembered of increasing the comprehensibility of material (Ley *et al.*, 1972; Bradshaw *et al.*, 1975). The findings of these experiments which are

Table 9. *Summary of studies of recall of medical information varying in comprehensibility as measured by the Flesch Formula*

Investigators	Material	Difficulty	Recalled %
Ley *et al.* (1972)	(*a*) X-ray leaflet	Easy	73 (ns)
		Hard	78
	(*b*) X-ray leaflet	Easy	79 ($p < 0.01$)
		Hard	59
Bradshaw *et al.* (1975)	Diet instructions		
	(*a*) Experiment 1	Easy	31 ($p < 0.25$)
		Hard	24
	(*b*) Experiment 2	Easy	43 ($p < 0.05$)
		Hard	25
	(*c*) Experiment 3	Easy	40 ($p < 0.01$)
		Hard	27

summarized in Table 9 show that in most cases recall can be increased by simplifying material.

The second method investigated was the use of a technique called 'explicit categorization'. This was based on the finding that clustering of items is associated with greater recall, for reviews see Jung (1968) and Cofer (1972). It was hypothesized that if medical information could be clustered for patients they should recall more of it. The method consists of the clinician providing clusters or categories of information and category names to go with them. Thus he says to the patient:

> I am going to tell you: what is wrong.
> what the treatment will be.
> what tests will be necessary.
> what you must do to help yourself.
> what the outcome will be.
> Now, first, what is wrong with you ....
> Secondly, what the treatment will be .... etc.

An analogue study showed that this technique increased recall in volunteers from six to nine out of fifteen fictitious medical statements

Table 10. *Mean proportions of information recalled by patients in the normal and explicit categorization conditions*

| | Mean proportions recalled | | |
	Diagnosis	Advice	Other information
Normal presentation	0·605	0·283	0·461
Explicit categorization	0·667	0·654	0·703

and the experiment was then repeated in a general practice situation. Once more it led to significant increases in recall (Ley *et al.*, 1973). The results for these patients are shown in Table 10.

The third technique is repetition. It is clear that the clinician could say everything twice to the patient in the time taken by explicit categorization. Unpublished analogue experiments have shown that repetition leads to increases in recall of the same magnitude as explicit categorization. Which of the two should be used is up to the clinician, although arguably the explicit categorization technique flows more smoothly.

The last technique was discovered by accident. It was noticed during studies of laymen's views of the importance of different types of medical statement that where a specific and a general version of a similar instruction were rated, the specific version was considered the more important. Thus, the statement 'You must lose weight' was considered less important than the statement 'You must lose half a stone in weight' and so on.

It had already been demonstrated that perceived importance is a determinant of memory, so it seemed reasonable to explore the possibility that specific advice would be better recalled than general advice. Bradshaw *et al.* (1975) conducted appropriate experiments and found that this was so. Their results are shown in Table 11.

Increasing patients' satisfaction with communications

At this stage in the research programme it had been demonstrated that failures of comprehension and memory were likely to be in part responsible for patients' dissatisfaction with communications and non-compliance.

It was therefore necessary to apply the findings to the improvement of communications. As a first step an attempt was made to increase patients' satisfaction with communications in the hospital situation.

Table 11. *Differences in recall of specifically and generally phrased instructions about dieting*

Subjects	Mean percentage recalled	
	General	Specific
1. Volunteer subjects given *both* specific and general statements to recall	10·2	45
2. Volunteer subjects given *either* specific *or* general statements	19·0	49
3. Obese women given *either* specific *or* general statements	16·0	51

Three groups of medical in-patients were studied. The control group received the hospital's normal procedure. In the experimental group patients received an extra visit from the doctor once every ten days or so, in which he tried to ensure that they had understood what they had already been told. No new topics were introduced, and the interview was restricted to simply increasing understanding of information already given. Visits lasted less than five minutes. As the extra medical attention might in itself have affected satisfaction a placebo group was also studied. Patients in this group also received extra visits from the doctor every ten days or so, but the interviews were concerned with how the patient was settling in, privacy, noise, food, and other such topics.

A detailed description of the experiment which involved a fairly complex design to counterbalance differences between wards and times of year is given by Ley *et al.* (1976). The results of the experiment showed that increases in understanding led to significantly greater satisfaction with communications. Eighty per cent of the experimental group were satisfied with the communications aspect of their hospital stay as opposed to 41 per cent of the placebo group and 48 per cent of the controls.

It should, perhaps, be pointed out, that satisfaction with communications is likely to be justified on practical as well as humanitarian grounds. Satisfied patients are reported to be more compliant by Freemon *et al.* (1971) and Kincey *et al.* (1975).

Increasing patients' compliance with advice

Effects of increasing comprehension and/or memory. Two experiments
have been carried out to see the effects of increasing comprehension
and memory on compliance.

Ley, Jain, and Skilbeck (1974) attempted to increase the accuracy
with which psychiatric out-patients took their medication. Interviews
with patients suggested that patients often did not realize that their
medicine might take some time to produce effects, and that they did
not know what to do if they forgot to take a tablet.

Accordingly a brief leaflet was prepared which gave information
on these topics for patients receiving anti-depressants and for patients
receiving tranquillizers. Three versions of each leaflet were prepared
which differed in Reading Ease as measured by the Flesch Formula.
One was hard, one moderately hard, and one easy. Eighty consecutive
new out-patients who received either anti-depressant drugs alone or
tranquillizers alone were assigned randomly to receiving one of the
three versions of the leaflet, or no leaflet. Patients received a prescription for their medicine and were asked to bring any remaining tablets
with them on their return visit approximately three weeks after their
initial visit. The tablets were then counted and an error score worked
out. This was the difference between the number of tablets which
should have been taken and the number which were taken, as a
percentage of the number which should have been taken. Mean error
scores for the various groups of patients are shown in Table 12.

The second investigation used obese women as subjects. The obese
were chosen as subjects for our compliance studies because it was
necessary to have a condition of some clinical interest where: (1) there

Table 12. *The effects of providing information leaflets
varying in difficulty to depressed and anxious patients*

Type of leaflet	Mean differences between tablets taken and tablets prescribed as a percentage of tablets prescribed	
	Depressed patients	*Anxious patients*
Easy	2·7	5·8
Moderately difficult	8·1	7·8
Difficult	14·5	14·9
No leaflet	16·2	14·6

Table 13. *Weight loss in groups receiving ordinary or experimental (super-memory) leaflet*

	Mean weight loss in pounds at			
	2 weeks	*4 weeks*	*8 weeks*	*16 weeks*
Ordinary leaflet	2·7	4·7	7·7	8·2
Experimental leaflet	4·4	8·6	12·3	15·4

were adequate numbers of subjects, and (2) there was an objective criterion of compliance (ie weight loss).

In this experiment two versions of a leaflet designed to motivate and persuade women to start and keep to a low carbohydrate diet were prepared. Both versions contained the same content. The control version was moderately easy according to the Flesch Formula. The other version was very easy, and contained explicit categorization and repetition. It should, therefore, have been easier to understand and remember.

Obese subjects who had answered newspaper and television appeals for volunteers were assigned at random to receiving one or other versions of the leaflet. In addition all subjects received an identical low carbohydrate diet guide. This written material was the only persuasive and technical information given to subjects, except that specific queries about the diet schedule were answered at follow-up visits. Subjects were followed up for sixteen weeks with the results shown in Table 13.

The experimental leaflet produced significantly more weight loss than the control leaflet. Thus attempts to increase patients' comprehension and/or memory for advice can result in gains in compliance in the areas of medicine taking and dieting.

Effects of social psychological variables. It was stated earlier that if patients understood and remembered all of the advice given to them it would be unlikely that there would then be complete compliance. Comprehension and memory are necessary but not sufficient causes of compliance. Other factors need to be investigated in attempts to increase compliance.

Social psychologists have discovered a number of variables and procedures which appear to facilitate attitude change (for reviews see Berscheid and Walster, 1969, and Kiesler *et al.*, 1969). Ley and Spelman (1967) suggested that many of these might be applied to the problem of patient compliance with medical advice. The ones they advocated were: (1) use of group decision procedures; (2) use of two-sided communications; (3) correct use of fear-arousing appeals.

Group decision procedures were invented and studied by Kurt Lewin and his associates in the 1940s and 1950s (Lewin, 1954). In the group decision procedure there is a discussion of the problems involved in following the advice; the discussion is detached, ie, in terms of subjects like themselves; the members of the group have to make a decision; the members of the group then have to publicly commit themselves to their decision. It is clear that this is a complicated package but while there is dispute about which of the variables involved is important (Bennett, 1955; Pennington *et al.*, 1958), the package seems to produce more reported compliance than the use of straight lecture procedures. This is true even in the two-person situation where the expert 'lectures' to one client or patient (Lewin, 1954). It is thus of potential use in any condition where there are sufficient numbers of patients available to form groups.

When advice is given to patients they are likely to be exposed to counter-propaganda, that is comments on the advice and conflicting advice which militate against the original advice being accepted. The effectiveness of such counter-propaganda can be reduced by the use of two-sided communications which not only present the case for following the advice but also deal with the case against it (Hovland *et al.*, 1949). Although two-sided communications are less effective initially the resistance to counter-propaganda that they induce should make them better bets at producing compliance in the long term. Where counter-propaganda is met one would therefore predict an interaction between the sidedness of a communication and the passage of time in producing compliance.

There is considerable dispute about the effectiveness of fear arousal in producing compliant behaviour and attitude change (Janis, 1967; Leventhal, 1970). Briefly and doing scant justice to these theorists, Janis expects curvilinear relationship between degree of fear arousal and compliance, while Leventhal expects linear ones. However, there is agreement that different levels of fear arousal can be expected to produce different effects.

To assess the usefulness of these variables in a quasi-medical situation two sets of experiments have been conducted with obese women. The first set of these is described by Ley *et al.* (1974*b*) and the second set by Skilbeck *et al.* (1976) and Tulips *et al.* (1974). These

Table 14. *Social psychological variables and compliance*

	Mean weight loss in pounds at 8 weeks	
Group	1st series	2nd series
Group decision	9·06	—
Lecture	7·69	—
Low fear arousal	6·75	13·7
Medium fear arousal	8·10	11·0
High fear arousal	7·69	12·0
One-sided communications	6·25	11·9
Two-sided communications	8·63	12·8

experiments have involved comparisons of group decision and lecture procedures, one- and two-sided communications, and three levels of fear arousal. None of these variables had had any effect on compliance as assessed by weight loss.

The results of these two series of experiments are shown in Table 14. As well as there being no over-all difference between one- and two-sided communications the possible interaction between sidedness of communication and time was not found either.

A number of explanations for these negative results can be proposed. Amongst them are the possibilities that the attitude change variables could not increase our subject's motivation because it was already at its peak, or that these variables affect attitudes but not behaviour. These possibilities are currently being investigated. It has also been found in our studies that the effects of fear will vary with the position of the fear appeal, and the subject's frequency of exposure to it (Skilbeck *et al.*, 1976). Indeed all of these variables will need to be investigated in greater detail and with greater refinement, but as the results stand they suggest that it is not possible at this stage to give clinicians easy, uncomplicated rules for the use of these variables.

Finally, a start has been made on the investigation of situational variables. Tulips *et al.* (1974) report on experimental attempts to increase compliance with a dietary regime amongst obese women by manipulating group cohesiveness. Two sets of subjects were assigned randomly to membership of nominal or cohesive groups. The cohesive group always attended together, were referred to as a group, were given name badges and were given a group target. The nominal

Table 15. *Mean weight loss in cohesive and control groups*

| | *Mean weight loss in pounds at* | | | |
	2 weeks	*4 weeks*	*8 weeks*	*16 weeks*
Control groups	4·9	6·5	9·0	11·0
Cohesive groups	5·8	8·0	12·6	19·8

Control versus cohesive groups: $p < 0.001$

groups attended together at the first session but no steps were taken to keep them together as a group. They might or might not meet at follow-up sessions and none of the special cohesiveness enhancing measures were taken. Members of the cohesive groups lost significantly more weight than the controls. The results are shown in Table 15.

Conclusion

Using a very simple model it has proved possible to account for much of the variance in patient compliance and satisfaction with communication. It has also proved possible to obtain worthwhile improvements in both of these areas. Patients' lack of understanding and forgetting complicated by diffidence resulting in lack of requests for enlightenment, seem to be major factors in patients' dissatisfaction with communications. It has already been suggested that the reduction of patients' diffidence should produce not only more patient satisfaction, but also, by providing feedback to the clinician improve his communicative skills. A series of investigations to find ways of reducing patients' diffidence, and to assess the effects of this on patient satisfaction, and clinicians' communicative behaviour would be well worth pursuing.

Even with high levels of comprehension and memory amongst patients some will remain dissatisfied with communication and many will remain non-compliant. To deal with these problems satisfactorily more complicated models will be necessary. However, even before such models have been developed, it should be possible to effect some improvements by applying social psychological findings to the clinical field, as in the experiment on group cohesiveness and weight loss.

There is also a great deal of tidying up research to be done. For example, does explicit categorization work with all possible sets of categories? Are some sets better than others? Can patients be trained to categorize for themselves? Why does a decrease in difficulty of material sometimes lead to increased recall and sometimes not?

Finally, the principles established so far lend themselves to application in other areas, and it would be interesting to see if they lead to significant gains in the health education field.

References

BENNETT, E. B. (1955). 'Discussion, decision, commitment and concensus in group decision', *Human Relations*, **8**, 251–73.

BERSCHEID, E., and WALSTER, E. (1969). 'Attitude change', in Mills, J. (ed.), *Experimental Social Psychology* (London: Collier-Macmillan).

BOYLE, C. M. (1970). 'Differences between patients' and doctors' interpretation of some common medical terms', *Br. med. J.* **2**, 286–9.

BRADSHAW, P. W., LEY, P., KINCEY, J. A., and BRADSHAW, J. (1975). 'Recall of medical advice: comprehensibility and specificity', *Br. J. soc. clin. Psychol.* **14**, 55–62.

CARSTAIRS, V. (1970). *Channels of Communication* (Edinburgh: Scottish Home and Health Department).

CARTWRIGHT, A. (1964). *Human Relations and Hospital Care* (London: Routledge and Kegan Paul).

CATTELL, R. B. (1973). *Personality and Mood by Questionnaire* (San Francisco: Josey-Bass).

CENTRAL HEALTH SERVICES COUNCIL (1963). *Communication between Doctors, Nurses and Patients* (London: HMSO).

COFER, C. N. (1972). 'Properties of verbal materials and verbal learning', in Kling, J. W., and Riggs, L. A. (eds), *Woodworth and Schlosberg's 'Experimental Psychology'* (London: Methuen).

DAVIS, M. S. (1968a). 'Physiologic, psychological and demographic factors in patient compliance with doctor's orders', *Medical Care*, **6**, 115–22.

—— (1968b). 'Variations in patients' compliance with doctors' advice: an empirical analysis of patterns of communication', *Am. J. Publ. Hlth*, **58**, 274–88.

DEPARTMENT OF HEALTH AND SOCIAL SECURITY (1973). *Report of the Committee on Hospital Complaints Procedure* (London: HMSO).

FLESCH, R. (1948). 'A new readability yardstick', *J. Appl. Psychol.* **32**, 221–33.

FLETCHER, C. M. (1973). *Communication in Medicine*. Rock Carling Monograph (London: Nuffield Provincial Hospitals Trust).

FRANCIS, V., KORSCH, B., and MORRIS, M. (1969). 'Gaps in doctor–patient communication: patients' response to medical advice', *New Engl. Med. J.* **280**, 535–40.

FREEMON, B., NEGRETE, V. F., DAVIS, M., and KORSCH, B. M. (1971). 'Gaps in doctor–patient communication: doctor–patient interaction analysis', *Pediat. Res.* **5**, 298–311.

HILDRETH, H. M. (1946). 'A battery of feeling and attitude scales for clinical use', *J. Clin. Psychol.* **6**, 214–21.

HOUGHTON, H. (1968). 'Problems in hospital communication: an experimental study', in McLachlan, G. (ed.), *Problems and Progress in Medical Care: Essays on Current Research*. Third Series (Oxford University Press for the Nuffield Provincial Hospitals Trust).

HOVLAND, C. I., LUMSDAINE, A. A., and SHEFFIELD, F. D. (1949). 'The effects of presenting "one-side" versus "both sides" in changing opinions on a controversial subject', in *Studies in Social Psychology in World War II*, vol. iii (Princeton, New Jersey: University of Princeton Press).

HUGH-JONES, P., TANSER, A. R., and WHITBY, C. (1964). 'Patient's view of admission to a London teaching hospital', *Br. med. J.* 2, 660–4.

JANIS, I. L. (1967). 'Effects of fear arousal on attitude change: Recent developments in theory and experimental research', in Berkowitz, L. (ed.), *Advances in Experimental Social Psychology* (New York: Academic Press).

JERSILD, A. (1929). 'Primacy, recency, frequency and vividness', *J. Exper. Psychol.* 12, 58–70.

JOYCE, C. R. B., CAPLE, G., MASON, M., REYNOLDS, E., and MATHEWS, J. A. (1969) 'Quantitative study of doctor–patient communication', *Q. Jl Med.* 38, 183–94.

JUNG, J. (1968). *Verbal Learning* (New York: Holt, Rinehart and Winston).

KIESLER, C. A., COLLINS, B. C., and MILLER, N. (1969). *Attitude Change* (New York: Wiley).

KINCEY, J., BRADSHAW, P. W., and LEY, P. (1975). 'Satisfaction and reported acceptance of advice in general practice: a preliminary study', *Jl R. Coll. Gen. Practit.* 25, 558–66.

KORSCH, B., GOZZI, E., and FRANCIS, V. (1968). 'Gaps in doctor–patient communications: doctor–patient interaction and patient satisfaction', *Pediatrics*, 62, 855–61.

LEVENTHAL, H. (1970). 'Findings and theory in the study of fear communications', in Berkowitz, L. (ed.), *Advances in Experimental Social Psychology*, 4, 11–19, 186 (New York: Academic Press).

LEWIN, K. (1954). 'Studies in group decision', in Cartwright, D., and Zander, A., *Group Dynamics* (London: Tavistock Publications).

LEY, P. (1972a). 'Complaints made by hospital staff and patients: a review of the literature', *Bull. Br. Psychol. Soc.* 25, 115–20.

—— (1972b). 'Comprehension, memory and the success of communications with the patient', *J. Inst. Hlth Educ.* 10, 23–9.

—— (1972c). 'Primacy, rated importance and the recall of medical information', *J. Hlth Soc. Behav.* 13, 311–17.

—— (1973). 'The measurement of comprehensibility', *J. Inst. Hlth Educ.* 11, 17–20.

—— (1974). 'Communication in the clinical setting', *Br. J. Orthodont.* 1, 173–7.

—— GOLDMAN, M., BRADSHAW, P. W., KINCEY, J. A., and WALKER, C. M. (1972). 'The comprehensibility of some X-ray leaflets', *J. Inst. Hlth Educ.* 10, 47–55.

—— BRADSHAW, P. W., EAVES, D. E., and WALKER, C. M. (1973). 'A method for increasing patients recall of information presented to them', *Psychol. Med.* 3, 217–20.

—— —— KINCEY, J., and ATHERTON, S. T. (1976). 'Increasing patients' satisfaction with communications', *Br. J. soc. clin. Psychol.* (in press).

—— —— —— COUPER-SMARTT, J., and WILSON, M. (1974). 'Psychological variables in weight control', in Burland, W. L., Samuel, P. D., and Yudkin, J. (eds), *Obesity 1974* (London: Churchill).

—— JAIN, V. K., and SKILBECK, C. E. (1974). 'An attempt to reduce patients' medication errors by the provision of information leaflets' (unpublished manuscript).

—— and SPELMAN, M. S. (1965). 'Communications in an out-patient setting', *Br. J. soc. clin. Psychol.* 4, 114–16.

—— —— (1967). *Communicating with the Patient* (London: Staples Press).

LOVIUS, J., LOVIUS, B. B. J., and LEY, P. (1973). 'Comprehensibility of the literature given to children at a dental hospital', *J. Publ. Hlth Dent.* 33, 23–26.

MCGHEE, A. (1961). *The Patient's Attitude to Nursing Care* (Edinburgh: Livingstone).

PENNINGTON, D. F., HARAREY, F., and BASS, B. M. (1958). 'Some effects of decision and discussion on coalescence, change and effectiveness', *J. Appl. Psychol.* 42, 404–8.

POSTMAN, L. (1972). 'Transfer interference and forgetting', in Kling, J. W., and Riggs, L. A. (eds), *Woodworth and Schlosberg's 'Experimental Psychology'* (London: Methuen).

RAPHAEL, W. (1967). 'Do we know what patients think? A survey comparing the view of patients, staff and committee members', *Internat. J. Nurs. Stud.* 4, 209–23.

—— (1969). *Patients and their Hospitals* (London: King Edward's Fund).

ROTH, P. M., CARON, M. S., ORT, R. S., BERGER, D. G., ALBEE, G. W., and STREETER, G. A. (1962). 'Patients' beliefs about peptic ulcer and its treatment', *Annals Intern. Med.* 56, 72–80.

SKILBECK, C. E., TULIPS, J. G., and LEY, P. (1976). 'The effects of fear arousal, fear position, fear exposure, and sidedness on compliance with dietary instructions', *European J. Soc. Psychol.* (in press).

SPELMAN, M. S., and LEY, P. (1966). 'Knowledge of lung cancers and smoking habits', *Br. J. soc. clin. Psychol.* 5, 207–10.

—— —— and JONES, C. C. (1966). 'How do we improve doctor–patient communication in our hospitals', *World Hospitals*, 2, 126–9.

TULIPS, J. G., LEY, P., and SKILBECK, C. E. (1974). 'Further studies of psychological variables in weight control' (unpublished manuscript).

UNITED MANCHESTER HOSPITALS (1970). *Patient Satisfaction Survey 1968–69.*

WILD, A. A., and EVANS, J. (1968). 'The patient and the X-ray department', *Br. med. J.* 2, 607–9.

Persuasive communication
A social-psychological perspective on factors influencing communication effectiveness

Martin Fishbein
Professor of Psychology
University of Illinois at
Urbana-Champaign

Persuasive communication

When I was first asked to contribute to the original seminar, I had little, if any, knowledge of the area of medical communication. Perhaps even more embarrassing, it was not until I received copies of the other papers to be presented that I realized that the main area of concern was with problems of face-to-face communications among doctors, nurses, and patients. Although I had conducted two studies that could conceivably be considered as studies of communication in medical settings, both studies were concerned with assessing the effectiveness of mass, rather than face-to-face communications. In the course of the day's discussion however, it became clear that many of the problems are similar to, or the same as, the problems that have been faced by social psychologists in their attempts to understand the processes of communication and persuasion.

Before considering these problems, however it may be useful to briefly consider the role of communication and persuasion in medicine. I am sure that doctors and nurses, like many other professionals, do not think that 'persuasion' is a part of their jobs. Yet every day, medical practitioners try to change patients' beliefs about their state of health, the meaning of various symptoms, or the consequences of taking (or not taking) a given medicine, of smoking, of dieting, etc. Similarly, they prescribe certain drugs or courses of action and attempt to provide information that will increase the likelihood that their patients will follow the prescription.

Unfortunately, the word persuasion has taken on a negative connotation and most people prefer to believe that the purpose of their communications is to inform rather than to persuade. However, it must be realized that informing another person always involves communicating some information, and the communicator hopes that the receiver will accept the information, that the receiver will believe what he is told. To put this somewhat differently, the communicator hopes that the information he provides will produce a change in some of the receiver's beliefs. More often, the communicator also assumes that these changes in beliefs will have additional effects, such as reducing the receiver's anxieties or increasing the likelihood that the receiver will select the right course of action.

If the purpose of a communication is to change beliefs, feelings, or behaviours, then, whether we are prepared to admit it or not, we are involved in the communication and persuasion process. Persuasion need not be a dirty word; theoretically at least, it merely refers to the effects of a communication. If we want patients to give us more (or different kinds of) information about their health, or if we want them to follow certain recommendations, it is usually necessary to provide them with information that will increase the likelihood they will do so. Similarly, if a doctor wants a nurse to behave in certain ways (either in general, in certain situations, or with respect to a particular patient) the doctor must communicate this to the nurse: he must provide her with information that will influence her behaviour. The questions of whether the information communicated is accepted and whether it leads to the desired change in behaviour are questions of communication and persuasion. That is, the study of communication and persuasion is concerned with understanding the problem of 'Who says what to whom with what effect?' It is precisely this question that social psychologists have been attempting to answer for more than thirty-five years. More specifically, they have been concerned with manipulating communicator variables (the who), message variables (the what), and audience variables (the to whom) in an attempt to understand their influence on various measures of reception and attitude change (the effect).

Unfortunately, this approach has not been terribly successful, and as recently as five years ago a cursory look at the communication literature would have shown that social psychology had relatively little to contribute to an understanding of the communication and persuasion process; the thousands of studies conducted had not yielded a single generalizable principle of effective communication that would be of use to the practising communicator. It now appears, however, that all of this research has not gone for nought, and in the past five years I think we have begun to learn from our mistakes and finally begun to make some major breakthroughs in our understanding of the communication and persuasion process. What I should like to do in this paper is to discuss some of these new insights in the hope that people interested in the study of medical communication can not only benefit from our progress but, more importantly, can avoid making the same mistakes all over again.

Perhaps our major mistake was a failure to recognize that beliefs, attitudes, intentions, and behaviours are four very different variables with different determinants and with stable and systematic relations among them. Until very recently, the term attitude was used in a generic sense to refer not only to a person's affective feelings towards some object, but also to his cognitions (or beliefs) about the object and his conations (or behavioural intentions) with respect to the object. Thus although studies of communications and persuasion seemed similar in that they tested the effectiveness of a given communication or of a given manipulation (such as communicator credibility) by measuring the amount of attitude change produced, we can now see that some of these measures of attitude change were measures of belief, others were measures of attitudes, and still others were measures of intentions or behaviour.

A theoretical framework

A belief is a probability judgement that links some object or concept to some attribute.[1] The content of the belief is defined by the object and attribute in question, and the strength of the belief is defined by the person's subjective probability that the object–attribute relationship exists (or is true).

An attitude is a bipolar evaluative judgement of the object. It is essentially a subjective judgement that I like or dislike the object, that it is good or bad, that I'm favourable or unfavourable towards it.[2]

An intention is a probability judgement that links the individual to some action, and behaviour is an observable action that is quantifiable on either a dichotomous (ie he did/did-not perform action X) or a continuous scale (he donated £0 to £X to a charity).

Fig. 1 presents a brief summary of the relations between beliefs, attitudes, intentions, and behaviours with respect to a given object. From this it can be seen that a person holds many beliefs about any given object, that is, he associates that object with a variety of attributes. What we have found is that knowledge of a person's beliefs

1. The terms 'object' and 'attribute' are used in a generic sense and both terms may refer to any discriminable aspect of an individual's world. For example, I may believe that *Pill A* (an object) is *a depressant* (an attribute).
2. Once again, the term object is used in a generic sense. Thus I may have attitudes towards people, institutions, events, behaviours, outcomes, etc.

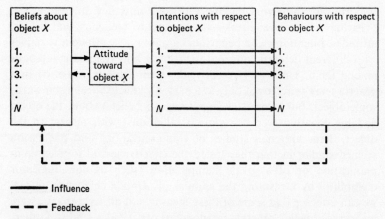

————— Influence

— — — Feedback

Fig. 1. *Schematic presentation of conceptual framework relating beliefs, attitudes, intentions, and behaviours with respect to a given object.*

about an object *and* his attitudes towards the associated attributes allow us to accurately predict his attitude towards the object *per se*. That is, it appears that a person's attitude towards any object is a function of his beliefs about that object. Notice however, that it is the *entire* set of beliefs that determines the attitude and *not* any single belief. As we shall see below, this is an important point because it implies that changing any one belief about an object may not change the person's attitude towards the object.

Once the person has formed an attitude he is predisposed (ie he intends) to perform a variety of behaviours with respect to, or in the presence of, the object. Once again, it must be noted that although his attitude does predispose him to perform a set of behaviours, it does not predispose him to perform any *specific* behaviour. This is perhaps the most important finding to come out of social psychology in the last ten years. By contrast to our previous assumption that changing a person's attitude towards some object would influence some particular behaviour with respect to that object, it is now clear that attitudes towards an object may have little or no influence on specific behaviours with respect to that object. Just as attitude is determined by the entire *set* of beliefs a person holds, the attitude only serves to predispose the person to engage in a *set* of behaviours that, when *taken together*, are consistent with the attitude.

This is really nothing more than a recognition of the fact that a person's attitude may be expressed in a variety of ways. For example, two people may like a third person equally well, but this does not mean that they will behave identically with respect to that person. There are various ways of expressing liking and one person may express it by inviting the person out for a drink, while this particular behaviour might never occur to the other person, perhaps because he is a teetotaller. However, the latter person might show his liking by inviting the person home for dinner. It has taken over fifty years to break down the fallacy of a one-to-one relation between attitudes and behaviours and, as we shall see below, the assumption of a one-to-one relationship has been one of the major factors impeding progress in understanding the communication process.

It is important to recognize however, that Fig. 1 does *not* imply that there is no relationship between attitude towards an object and intentions to engage in various behaviours with respect to that object. Indeed, it suggests that if one were interested in the totality of intentions a person held with respect to some object, knowledge of a person's attitude would be a useful predictor. That is, the more favourable the person's attitude, the more positive and the fewer negative behaviours he would intend to engage in. To put this somewhat differently, increasing a person's attitude towards some object should increase the *number* of positive behaviours he intends to engage in with respect to, or in the presence of that object. There is no guarantee however, that it will increase the person's intention to engage in any particular behaviour. Thus, for example, increasing a woman's attitude towards family planning might increase her intention to have a two-child family but not her intention to use contraceptives.

Finally, Fig. 1 also points out that a person's intention to engage in a specific behaviour with respect to an object is the primary determinant of that behaviour. That is, the single best predictor of whether or not a person will engage in a particular behaviour is his intention with respect to that behaviour. Unlike the relations between beliefs and attitudes, and attitude and intentions, we do assume a one-to-one relation between intention and behaviour. Thus, everything that was said about the attitude–intention relationship, also applies to the attitude–behaviour relationship. We can no longer assume that a person's attitude towards an object will be related to any specific behaviour the person engages in with respect to the object but it should be related to the pattern of behaviour he performs.

Unfortunately, most communications are not directed at changing patterns of behaviour, but are directed at some specific behaviour the communicator wants to change. As even the most cursory glance at the communication and persuasion literature will show, most communications appear to have been notoriously unsuccessful in producing behaviour change. The above analysis provides several explanations for this. First, most communications are based on the assumption that changing a person's attitude towards some object will change some specific behaviour towards that object. The above analysis points out that even if the communication were successful in producing a change in attitude, this may have little or no effect on the particular behaviour the communicator was interested in. Second, most attempts to change attitudes are based on the assumption that this can be done by changing one or more of the person's beliefs about the object. Here too, even if the communication were successful in changing those beliefs it was directed at, this is no guarantee that the person's attitude would change, since the attitude is based on the entire set of beliefs about the object that the person holds and not just the one or two beliefs attacked in the message. As we shall see below, changing one belief about an object may have unexpected impact effects on other beliefs about the object that the individual holds. Indeed, in many cases, although the communication may be effective in changing those beliefs it was directed at, the impact effect of the message on other beliefs about the object may actually serve to *lower*, rather than to raise, a person's attitude towards the object.

Before turning to a consideration of such message effects, however, it is necessary to consider those variables that are related to specific behaviours and intentions. In Fig. 2 it can again be seen that the immediate determinant of any given behaviour is the person's intention to engage in that behaviour. Two major variables have been found to serve as the determinants of an intention: (1) the person's attitude towards *performing the behaviour in question* and (2) his subjective norm with respect to performing the behaviour, that is, his subjective judgement that most people who are important to him think he should or should not engage in the behaviour. Please notice that this statement is not very profound; it would be surprising indeed if people did not intend to perform those behaviours that (1) they themselves evaluated positively or (2) important others thought they should perform. What is interesting however, is that the relative weights of these determinants vary as a function of the behaviour in question and individual difference variables. For some behaviours

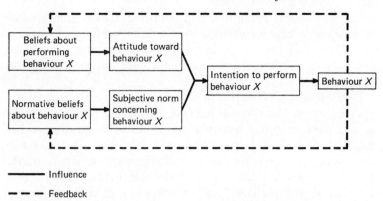

Fig. 2. *Schematic presentation of conceptual framework for the prediction of specific intentions and behaviours.*

the person's intention is based almost entirely on his attitude towards performing the behaviour and little or no attention is paid to the prescriptions of important others. For other behaviours, the intention may be based primarily on the prescriptions of important others, and the person's attitude towards the behaviour has little or no influence. Similarly, some people (such as authoritarians) may place more weight on normative influences, while others (such as introverts) may place more weight on attitudinal considerations.

Even at this relatively global level, several important points can be made. First, a relatively simple shift in focus from the object the behaviour is directed towards to the behaviour *per se*, again places importance upon attitude as a predictor of behaviour. So all the research done with respect to attitudes towards objects has not been in vain, for all of the findings can also be applied to understanding, measuring, and changing attitudes towards behaviours. From a theoretical perspective, an attitude is an attitude, and it makes little or no difference if we are talking about attitudes towards people, institutions, events, or behaviours. That is, as can be seen in Fig. 2 (and similar to Fig. 1), a person's attitude towards performing a given behaviour is viewed as a function of his beliefs about performing the behaviour (just as his attitude towards an object was viewed as a function of his beliefs about the object). Thus, just as we may change a person's attitude towards an object by changing the *set* of beliefs the person holds about that object, so too can we change a person's attitude towards performing a given behaviour by changing the *set* of his beliefs about performing that behaviour. However, it can also be seen that even if a communication were successful in changing a person's attitude towards the behaviour in question, this, again, does not necessarily guarantee change in his intention to perform the behaviour.

Recall that some behavioural intentions are primarily under normative control, and if this is the case, changing a person's attitude towards performing the behaviour will have little or no effect on his intention. Indeed, in such a situation, behavioural intentions will only change if one is successful in changing the subjective norm. Fig. 2 also indicates that the subjective norm (like attitudes) is a function of other beliefs. More specifically, a person's judgement that 'most people who are important to me think I should/should not perform this behaviour' is viewed as a function of his *normative beliefs*, that is, his beliefs that specific referents (be they individuals or groups) think he should or should not engage in the behaviour, weighted by his motivation to comply with these referents. Here too, it should be noted that the subjective norm is a function of the *set* of normative beliefs the person holds, and it is not necessarily related to any single normative belief. Thus, changing a person's belief that a particular referent thinks he should (or should not) engage in the behaviour may not influence his subjective norm: that is his judgement that 'most people who are important to me' think I should (or should not) perform the behaviour.

For those of you who are quantitatively oriented, I should perhaps mention that all of the above statements can be put in mathematical form. More specifically, the relations in Fig. 1 can be described as follows:

$$\sum_{}^{n} b_i e_i \approx A_o \approx \sum_{}^{n} I_i e_i \approx \sum_{}^{n} B_i e_i.$$

Where b_i = the strength of belief i about concept o, ie, the subjective probability that concept o is related to some attribute i.
A_o = the person's attitude towards concept o.
I_i = the strength of intention i with respect to concept o, ie, the subjective probability that the person intends to perform some behaviour i with respect to concept o.
B_i = the actual performance or non-performance of behaviour i.

e_i = the subject's evaluation of (or attitude towards) attribute
i or behaviour i.

n = the number of salient beliefs the subject holds about
concept o or the number of intentions or behaviours
that could be performed with respect to concept o.

The $\approx$ sign indicates that we are dealing with functional or causal
relationships and *not* identities. That is, attitudes are functionally related to (or determined by) a person's beliefs and his evaluations of
associated attributes; the attitude however, is *not* the beliefs and
evaluations. Further, describing the relationships quantitatively
makes it clear that changing one or two beliefs about an object
may not change the person's attitude towards the object. That is,
attitude is viewed as a function of $\sum b_i e_i$, and it is only when this
value changes that one can expect a change in attitude. Thus, although a message may change a particular belief that it is directed
at, it may also have impact effects on other beliefs and the total set
of changes may produce a $\sum b_i e_i$ score that is identical to the original
$\sum b_i e_i$ score. If this were the case, then even though there were considerable changes in beliefs, no change in attitude would be expected.

Similarly, although it can be seen that an increase in attitude
should produce an increase in the value of $\sum I_i e_i$ and $\sum B_i e_i$, the
mathematical expression makes it clear that it is impossible to state
which particular intentions or behaviours will be affected.

The relations in Fig. 2 can be described as follows:

$$B \approx I \approx [(A_{act})w_1 + (SN)w_2] \approx \left[(\sum_{i=1}^{n} b_i e_i) \; w_1 + (\sum_{j=1}^{n} N_j m_j) \; w_2 \right].$$

Where B = the performance or non-performance of behaviour x.

I = the intention to perform behaviour x.

A_{act} = the attitude towards performing behaviour x.

SN = the subjective norm concerning the performance of behaviour x, ie, the person's subjective judgement that
'most people who are important' to him think he
should (or should not) perform behaviour x.

b_i = belief i about performing behaviour x, ie, the subjective probability that performing behaviour x will
lead to (or block) outcome i.

e_i = the evaluation of (or attitude towards) outcome i.

N_j = a normative belief concerning the performance of behaviour x, ie, the person's subjective judgement that

referent j thinks he should (or should not) perform behaviour x.

$m_j = $ the person's motivation to comply with referent j, ie,
the degree to which the person wants to do (or wants
to do the opposite of) what referent j thinks he should
do.

$n = $ the number of salient beliefs the subject holds about
performing behaviour x or the number of referents
relevant to the performance of behaviour x.

w_1 and $w_2 = $ empirically derived weights referring to the relative
strength of the two components in determining the
person's intention to perform behaviour x.

Once again, describing these relationships mathematically should
make it clear that changing a given belief about performing a specific
behaviour may not change the person's attitude towards performing
the behaviour (that is attitude is a function of $\sum b_i e_i$) and similarly,
changing a specific normative belief (for example, my doctor thinks
I should take one of these pills every night) may not change the
person's subjective norm (for example, most people who are important to me think I should not take one of these pills every night).
That is, similar to attitudes, the subjective norm is viewed as a function of the *set* of normative beliefs $(\sum N_j m_j)$, and it is only when this
value changes that a change in the subjective norm can be expected.
Further, it can also be seen that even if one were successful in changing a given attitude or a subjective norm, this does not guarantee a
change in intention. Once again, the intention is seen as a function
of both the attitudinal and normative components *and* their relative
weights (ie, of $[(A_{act})w_1 + (SN)w_2]$) and it is only when the value of
this expression changes that a change in intention can be expected.
Clearly, if either the attitudinal or normative component carries little
or no weight in the determination of the intention (ie, if w_1 or w_2
have values close to zero), changing that component will not change
the value of the expression.

Finally, it should be noted that Figs 1 and 2, as well as their
mathematical representations, imply a causal chain linking beliefs
to attitudes, attitudes (and beliefs) to intentions, and intentions to
behaviours. It should be clear that one does not change attitudes,
intentions, or behaviours directly, but only by changing beliefs that
are functionally related to these variables. Thus, for example, if I

wish to change some specific behaviour, I would have to change the person's intention to perform that behaviour. In order to do this however, I would either have to change his attitude towards performing the behaviour or his subjective norm concerning the behaviour. Which of these two I would attack would depend upon their relative weights in determining the intention. However, in order to change either the attitude or the subjective norm, I must ultimately fall back on changing beliefs; either beliefs that performing the behaviour will lead to certain outcomes (to change the attitude), or normative beliefs about the prescriptions of revelant others (to change the subjective norm)[1].

Indeed, change in any attitude, be it towards an object, person, institution, event or a behaviour, ultimately rests on changing the beliefs underlying the attitude. This is important, because it points out that in large part, the effectiveness of any communication will depend upon its ability to produce changes in beliefs. It also points out that the success or failure of any communication will depend in large part upon its content and the degree to which that content is theoretically tied to the goal of the communication.

Message content

This brings us to the second major mistake that social psychologists and others have made in attempting to understand the communication process. I think it's fair to say that most people who have been interested in communication have paid little or no attention to the content of the message. Instead, they have been concerned with discovering variables that would increase or decrease the 'persuasiveness' of a given message, irrespective of its contents. For example, there have been literally hundreds of studies conducted to investigate the effects of 'communicator credibility'. Typically, the experimenter

---

1. It should be noted that attitudes can also be changed by changing the evaluation of associated attributes and that subjective norms can also be changed by changing the subject's motivation to comply with a specific referent. However, in both these cases, one must again ultimately change beliefs. That is, the evaluation of an associated attribute is nothing more than the person's attitude towards that attribute, and thus a change in this attitude will require changing beliefs about the attribute. Similarly, although the determinants of motivation to comply are still not well understood, it does seem clear that a person's motivation to comply with a given referent is some function of his beliefs about that referent and, in particular, beliefs about the referent's power, prestige, expertise, trustworthiness, etc.

constructs a message that he assumes will produce a change in some belief or attitude. In so doing he makes the assumption that if people believe the contents of this message, then they will also believe that X is Y, or that they will become more favourable to X. I will return to this point shortly; right now, however, let me merely point out that to the best of my knowledge, these assumptions underlying message construction have rarely been explicitly tested. Once the message has been constructed, the actual experiment is relatively straightforward: the same message is usually given to two groups of subjects; one group is told that the communicator is a 'high credibility source' (an expert) and the other is told the communicator is a 'low credibility source' (a charlatan). The two groups are then compared in terms of the amount of change the message produced in either the belief or the attitude. Although over all studies there is probably a slight tendency for more change to occur when the message is attributed to a 'high' rather than a 'low' credibility source, it is not at all uncommon to find that there are no differences between the groups, or even that the 'low' credibility source actually produced more change. Nowhere in this literature, however, is there even a suggestion that the amount of change produced might be some function of the content of the message, or that the differential effectiveness of high and low credibility communicators might depend, even in part, on the message content. Clearly, if the content of the message were unrelated to the belief or attitude being considered, then even if the message were accepted by more people who were told it came from a high credibility source, no differential changes in the belief or attitude would be expected. Similarly, if the investigator's assumption was wrong, ie, if there was a negative relation between acceptance of message content and the belief or attitude being considered, then, even if the high credibility source produced more acceptance, an analysis of belief or attitude change would suggest that the low credibility source produced more change in the dependent variable.

The main point to be made is that it is only when one starts to pay attention to message content, and in particular, to the relations between the message content and some specific dependent variable (be it a belief, attitude, intention, or behaviour), that one can start to understand the communication process. What we have already seen is that most messages are probably based on inappropriate and erroneous assumptions. We have tended to assume that changing one or two beliefs about some object would change some specific behaviour with respect to that object. What I want to point out is that although an individual may completely accept (ie believe) the contents of a given communication, the degree to which acceptance of this information will produce a change in some other belief, attitude, intention, or behaviour depends largely upon the theoretical links between the message content and the dependent variable in question.

False assumptions

Generally speaking, any communication can be viewed as a series of belief statements, ie, statements that link some object or concept to some attribute. Perhaps the first question to be asked is whether the belief statements comprising the message are identical to, or at least theoretically related to, the beliefs that one would have to change in order to produce changes in other beliefs, attitudes, intentions, or behaviours. What I have been trying to point out is that very different beliefs will have to be attacked depending upon the ultimate goal of the communication. For example, a message directed at changing a person's attitude towards some object will have to attack very different beliefs than a message directed at changing a person's intention to perform some specific behaviour with respect to that object. I honestly believe that if people were forced to be explicit about the particular assumptions they were making in constructing a communication, they would quickly realize that many of their assumptions were wrong. During discussion it has become clear that many of the failures in doctor–patient and patient–doctor or patient–nurse communications really occur because of assumptions made by the communicator. For example, a doctor may want his patient to believe that 'my doctor is really concerned with my welfare'. However, the doctor may not feel that he can simply tell the patient he is concerned with his welfare for various reasons: the patient will not believe it or it is too embarrassing. In such a case, the doctor may *assume* that he can communicate his concern by other, indirect means. He may assume that if he asks the patient about his family and his job, the patient will infer that the doctor is concerned with his welfare. Unfortunately, this assumption may not be right, and instead the patient might infer that 'the doctor is wasting a lot of time asking silly questions that have nothing to do with my problem'. In this case, rather than improving rapport with the patient, the doctor's communication may actually be harmful to the doctor–patient relationship. These same kinds of problems also enter into patient–doctor or patient–nurse interactions. For example, it appears that many patients are unwilling to simply tell a nurse that they are in pain. Thus, rather than directly saying, 'I am in pain', patients attempt to do this indirectly, for example, by seeking the nurse's attention by asking for a bedpan. Once again, the patient is making an assumption that 'if I ask the nurse for a bedpan, she will infer that I'm in pain'. Unfornately, in most cases, the nurse is not likely to make this inference, and instead she will probably do nothing more than bring the bedpan. Notice that in both cases the communicator's assumption is a relatively simple one: the communicator assumes that if he says A, the receiver will infer B.

By contrast to this, most persuasive communications involve a chain of assumptions linking changes in beliefs to changes in attitudes, changes in attitudes to changes in intentions, and changes in intentions to changes in behaviour. Even more important, most persuasive communications involve a different type of assumption, namely, the assumption that the entire chain of effects depends upon the receiver's acceptance of the message content. Most persuasive communications are based on the assumption that the persuasive effects of a message depend primarily on the degree to which the communicator accepts the contents of the message, ie, believes what the communicator tells him. This is perhaps the third major mistake that has been made by investigators of persuasive communication. While this assumption is true in part, it grossly oversimplifies the communication and persuasion process.

As was pointed out above, any communication can be viewed as a series of belief statements or 'source beliefs'. It now seems clear that if one wishes to understand the communication process, there are three different questions which must be asked with respect to a given belief statement: (1) Does the receiver accept the source belief, ie, does he believe (assign a high probability) to the statement contained in the message? (2) Is his post-exposure belief different than his pre-exposure belief? That is, did the receiver yield to the message content: did the message change the receiver's belief? (3) Did the source belief have an impact on other beliefs held by the receiver? To put this somewhat differently, it is now becoming clear that in order to be effective, a message must not only be *accepted*, but it must be *yielded to*. In addition, its effectiveness will depend in large part upon the degree to which it has unexpected or unanticipated *impact effects*.

In order to clarify these distinctions, let us consider a hypothetical example. Suppose that a doctor wants his patient to take a certain medicine, and he believes he can increase the chances of this occurring if he can convince the patient that 'taking these pills regularly will reduce your anxiety'. To put this somewhat differently, the doctor assumes that if he can get the patient to believe that 'taking these pills will reduce my anxiety' it will increase the likelihood that the patient will follow his prescription. Note first, that the doctor is assuming that the patient doesn't already hold this belief.

I think it is interesting that one of the major problems in many persuasive attempts is the communicator's failure to consider the kind and amount of information the receiver already has. All too often, a communicator fails to recognize that the receiver already holds the beliefs that comprise his message. In these cases, the receiver will accept the doctor's statement, but this acceptance does not produce a change. The patient may accept the doctor's statement, without yielding to it. If no change in this belief occurs (ie, if no yielding occurs) then clearly, even though the doctor's communication was accepted, no change in behaviour could be expected.

However, let us assume that the doctor was successful, ie, that following the communication, the patient was more certain that 'taking these pills will reduce my anxiety'. Theoretically, changing the belief about taking these pills could influence the receiver's attitude towards 'taking these pills'. In fact, implicitly or explicitly, the doctor had made the assumption that changing the belief about 'taking these pills' would produce a change in the patient's attitude towards 'taking these pills' and that this change in attitude would ultimately lead to the behavioural change. However, as we have already seen, the patient's attitude towards 'taking these pills' is not solely based upon his belief that 'taking these pills will reduce my anxiety', but on the entire set of beliefs he has about 'taking these pills'. This is important for it implies that if the doctor's statement had an impact on other beliefs about 'taking these pills' that the patient held, these impact effects would also influence the patient's attitude towards 'taking these pills'. What we have tended to ignore is the fact that changing one belief about a concept (such as 'taking these pills') will usually effect other beliefs the person holds about that concept. In the present case, if the patient came to believe that 'taking these pills will reduce my anxiety', he might also infer (ie, believe) that taking these pills will affect me in other ways: taking these pills will reduce my capacity to work, etc. If this were the case, then even though the doctor's communication were completely effective in terms of changing the belief it was directed at, the communication would have exactly the opposite effects on the subject's attitude towards taking the pills than the effects the doctor was trying to achieve. Rather than making the patient's attitude more favourable towards the pills, the communication may actually have achieved the reverse.

To summarize briefly then, I think we have made three major mistakes in our attempts to understand the process of communication and persuasion:

1. We have failed to distinguish between beliefs, attitudes, intentions, and behaviours.

2. We have failed to pay attention to message content, and particularly to the links between message content and the specific beliefs, attitudes, intentions, or behaviours we are trying to change.

3. We have failed to distinguish between *acceptance* of message content, *yielding* to message content, and the *impact* effects of the message.

A practical example

In order to illustrate these points, and also to demonstrate how these mistakes can be avoided, I'd like to describe briefly a recent study that was conducted by Dr Judy McArdle and myself. Dr McArdle had been working in an Alcoholic Treatment Unit (ATU) of a Veterans' Administration Hospital. Since only 50 per cent of the patients diagnosed as alcoholic were willing to be transferred to the ATU, Dr McArdle wished to increase this number, and she felt she could do it through the use of a persuasive communication. Her original idea was to send what is generally referred to as a 'fear appeal' message, ie, a message that points out the dangers of a given course of action, suggests how this action can be avoided, and recommends an alternative course of action. More specifically, she planned to send a message that (*a*) emphasized the negative consequences of continued drinking, (*b*) told the patients that they could gain control over their drinking by joining the ATU's programme, and (*c*) recommended that the receivers sign up for the Alcoholic Treatment Unit now.

Notice however, that from the point of view of the analysis given previously, such a message can only be of questionable effectiveness. According to the model presented above, if one wishes to increase the likelihood that a given person will sign up for the ATU, one must first change his intention to do so. In order to change this intention however, it is necessary to change either the person's attitude and/or his subjective norm about signing up for the ATU. Thus, the first question that must be asked is whether this particular behaviour is primarily under attitudinal or normative control. For the sake of argument, let us suppose that this particular behaviour is primarily under attitudinal control and, therefore, that it is necessary to change the person's attitude towards signing up for the ATU. According to our analysis, this can only be done by changing the person's beliefs. That is, in order to make him more favourable towards signing up, we have to provide him with information that will either increase his beliefs that signing up for the ATU will lead to positive consequences, or decrease his beliefs that signing up for the ATU will lead to negative consequences.[1]

Alternatively, we could try to convince him that 'Not signing up for the ATU' would lead to negative consequences and/or prevent the occurrence of positive consequences. The main point to be made however, is that if our analysis is correct, the message must change the receiver's beliefs about signing up or not signing up for the ATU if it is to be effective. Notice that in contrast to this, the fear appeal provides information about continued drinking, and although it does state that one can gain control over drinking by joining the ATU, it never directly attacks the receiver's beliefs about signing up for the ATU. At best, one can only hope that the receiver will infer that signing up for the ATU will prevent or that not signing up for the ATU will lead to the negative consequences of continued drinking described in the message. To put this somewhat differently, it appears that even if the fear appeal message were *accepted* and *yielded to*, it could only be effective in changing the receiver's behaviour if it had an impact effect on beliefs about signing. In contrast, one could design a communication that directly attacked the receiver's beliefs about signing up or not signing up for the ATU.

In order to test these notions, we constructed three persuasive messages. The first, which we called the traditional fear appeal, was

1. It would also be possible to increase his beliefs that signing up would prevent negative consequences.

exactly the message Dr McArdle originally had in mind. It was comprised of ten major belief statements each linking continued drinking with a different negative consequence (ie, a deterioration of physical health, a deterioration of relationships with your family: less freedom within the hospital, etc.). The message then argued that the ATU had a programme that could help them gain control over their drinking, and finally, it recommended that they 'sign up for the ATU now'. The second, which we called the negative appeal, was also comprised of ten major belief statements. Here however, each statement linked not signing up for the ATU with a different negative consequence. In fact, not signing up for the ATU was linked with the same ten negative consequences that appeared in the fear appeal message (ie, not signing up for the ATU will lead to a deterioration of your physical health; will lead to less freedom within the hospital, etc.). The negative message also ended with the recommendation to 'sign up for the ATU now'. The third message, which we called the positive message, was the mirror image of the negative message. It too was comprised of ten major belief statements, but each statement linked signing up for the ATU with a positive consequence. These consequences were the direct opposites of the negative consequences (ie, signing up for the ATU will improve your physical health; will give you more freedom within the hospital, etc.). Once again, the message also ended with a specific recommendation to 'sign up for the ATU now'.

Each message was presented to a different group of patients, half of whom had previously indicated willingness to sign up for the ATU and half of whom had previously refused to join. In addition, a fourth group served as a no-message control. The messages, each of which lasted about ten minutes, were tape-recorded by the director of the Alcoholic Treatment Unit. Immediately after hearing the message, the patients were given the opportunity of signing up for the programme. They were then asked to fill in some questionnaires which, among other things, allowed us to measure their beliefs about continued drinking, about signing up *and* not signing up for the ATU, and their attitudes towards continued drinking, signing up and not signing up. The results were as follows:

Acceptance of message content
The first question we asked concerned the degree to which the three messages were accepted by people receiving them. A direct measure

of *acceptance* of message content was built into the present study. More specifically, each message was comprised of ten basic source beliefs, with each statement linking the attitude object (ie signing up, not signing up, or continued drinking) to a positive or negative outcome. On the post-test, all subjects (including those in the no-message control) were asked to indicate the degree to which they personally believed each of these thirty statements. In Table 1 it can be seen that there were no significant differences between the groups in terms of the degree to which they accepted (believed) the ten statements comprising the particular message they received. Not unexpectedly, initially willing subjects were significantly more likely to believe the contents of the messages they received than were unwilling subjects ($X = 12.77$ vs 3.30, $P < 0.001$). There was, however, a significant interaction, since even subjects initially unwilling to be transferred to the ATU showed some acceptance of the fear message. Subjects who were initially unwilling to be transferred were likely to accept (believe) that continued drinking would lead to negative consequences.

Yielding to message content

Although the three messages were equally accepted, this cannot be taken as evidence that they produced equal amounts of change in corresponding beliefs, ie, that they were yielded to equally. Although no direct measure of change is available, yielding can be estimated by comparing the data presented in Table 1 with the corresponding data from the no message control group. Table 2 presents the mean

Table 1. *Acceptance of message content*

Subject type	Positive	Message condition Negative	Fear	Average
Willing	13·90	11·95	12·45	12·77
Unwilling	0·00	2·50	7·10	3·30
Over-all acceptance	6·95	7·23	9·78	

Source	df	MS	F
Type A	1	2745·63	65·17*
Condition B	2	97·06	2·30
$A \times B$	2	182·86	4·34†
Error	114	42·13	

*$P < 0.01$.   †$p < 0.05$.

estimates of the amount of change in beliefs comprising each message.
(ie the yielding) produced by the messages themselves.

Table 2. *Yielding to message content*

Subject type	Positive	Negative	Fear	Average
		Message condition		
Willing	3·55	5·70	1·15	3·47
Unwilling	0·80	6·95	1·60	3·12
Over-all yielding	2·17	6·35	1·38	

Cell entries represent differences between the experimental groups and appropriate controls. Only the differences in the negative conditions are significant.

Source	df	MS	F
Type *A*	1	3·68	0·09
Condition *B*	2	282·43	6·70*
A × *B*	2	44·80	1·06
Error	114	42·13	

*$p < 0.01$.

Over-all, the negative message was yielded to ($\overline{X} = 6.35$) to a
significantly greater extent than either the positive message ($\overline{X} = 2.17$)
or the fear appeal ($\overline{X} = 1.38$). Further, when one considers the
amount of change produced by each message, only the negative
message produced a significant amount of yielding. Somewhat
surprisingly, there was no over-all tendency for initially willing
subjects to yield more to the contents of the message they received
than initially unwilling subjects (3·47 vs 3·12). Although there was a
tendency for willing subjects to yield more to the contents of the
positive message than unwilling subjects, the interaction was not
significant. While these results indicate that only the negative message
was effective in changing the beliefs it contained, the messages may
also have impact effects.

Impact of the messages on non-mentioned beliefs

It should be recalled that underlying the use of a traditional fear
appeal message is the implicit assumption that respondents will make
inferences that signing up will lead to the ten positive consequences
and/or that not signing will lead to the ten negative consequences.
Along these same lines, the positive message could have an impact

Table 3. *Impact effects of the messages on primary beliefs*

(a) *Beliefs about signing*

	Message condition		
Subject type	Negative	Fear	Average
Willing	3·65	−1·65	1·00
Unwilling	6·45	−2·00	2·23
	5·04	−1·83	

Source	df	MS	F
Type *A*	1	41·09	1·73
Condition *B*	1	1266·11	53·31*
A × *B*	1	51·30	2·16
Error	76	23·75	

*p < 0·01.

(b) Beliefs about not signing

	Message condition		
Negative	Fear	Average	
3·80	−0·80	1·50	
0·85	−1·30	−0·23	
2·33	−1·05		

df	MS	F
1	37·46	1·41
1	1265·53	47·63*
1	24·44	0·92
76	26·57	

*p < 0·01.

on subjects' beliefs about not signing, and the negative message could have an impact about beliefs about signing.

Table 3 shows the impact effects of the messages on subjects' beliefs about signing up and not signing up for the ATU. In part (a) of Table 3 it can be seen that the negative appeal increased subjects' beliefs that signing up for the ATU would lead to positive consequences ($\overline{X} = +5·04$) while the fear appeal tended to decrease these beliefs ($\overline{X} = -1·83$). Similarly, in part (b) of Table 3, it can be seen that the positive appeal increased subjects' beliefs that not signing would lead to bad consequences ($\overline{X} = +2·33$) while the fear appeal tended to lower these beliefs ($\overline{X} = -1·05$). To put this somewhat differently, the positive and negative appeals produced positive impact effects. In marked contrast, even though there was little yielding to the traditional fear appeal, it did tend to have a negative impact on beliefs about signing up and not signing up for the ATU.

Over-all effect of the messages on beliefs

Table 4 presents the estimated change in all twenty beliefs (ten about signing up and ten about not signing up) produced by the three messages. Here it can be seen that over-all, both the positive and negative appeals had a significant positive effect on the total set of

Table 4. *Changes in all primary beliefs*

Subject type	Message condition			
	Positive	Negative	Fear	Average
Willing	7·35	9·35	−2·45	4·75
Unwilling	1·65	13·40	−3·30	3·92
Over-all change	4·50	11·37	−2·87	

Cell entries are differences between the experimental and control groups. All three over-all change scores are significant, ie, there is a significant difference between the experimental and control groups in each case.

Source	df	MS	F
Type A	2	20·83	0·11
Condition B	1	2031·46	10·91*
$A \times B$	2	237·66	1·28
Error	114	186·13	

*$p < 0.01$.

beliefs, while the fear appeal had a significant negative effect. Although there is no obvious explanation for this negative impact (or 'boomerang') effect of the traditional fear appeal message, this finding does make it clear that one cannot merely assume that inferences will be made that link a recommended course of action with avoidance of the dangers associated with a given state (for example, continued drinking). Indeed, rather than arriving at the appropriate inferences, the present study clearly indicates that subjects exposed to a message emphasizing the dangers associated with one course of action (ie, continued drinking) may actually infer that these dangers are *not* likely to be avoided by an alternative course of action (ie, signing up for the ATU) that is recommended in the message.

Effect of the message on the differential attitude towards signing

The implication of these differential belief changes can perhaps be seen most clearly in the next link in the chain of effects, ie, with respect to the respondent's differential attitudes towards the act of signing (ie, attitude towards signing up; attitude towards not signing up). Table 5 presents the mean change in differential attitudes of the respondents.

Table 5. *Changes in differential attitudes*

Subject type	Positive	Negative	Fear	Control	Average
			Message condition		
Willing	1·30	1·20	−0·80	0·50	0·55
Unwilling	0·40	1·15	−0·80	0·05	0·20
Over-all change	0·85	1·18	−0·80	0·28	

Source	df	MS	F
Type *A*	1	2·45	1·02
Condition *B*	3	15·04	6·24*
A × *B*	3	0·88	0·36
Error	152	2·41	

*$p < 0.01$.

While subjects in the no-message control did not change their attitudes over time, subjects receiving the positive and negative appeals significantly *increased* their differential attitudes towards signing while subjects receiving the traditional fear appeal significantly *decreased* their differential attitudes. According to our analysis, these changes in attitude should have influenced respondents' intentions to sign up for the ATU and thus their actual signing behaviour.

Effects of the messages on behaviour

Table 6 shows the proportion of signers in each condition. As expected, initially willing subjects were significantly more likely to sign (82·5 per cent) than those who were initially unwilling (13·7 per cent). In addition a significantly greater proportion of subjects exposed to the positive and negative appeals actually signed up for admission to the ATU than subjects exposed to the traditional fear appeal. More importantly, a significant interaction indicated the differential effectiveness of the various persuasive appeals. Considering only subjects who initially indicated that they were not willing to transfer to the ATU, none of those in the no-message control changed their

Table 6. *Percentage of respondents signing up for the ATU*
($N = 20$/cell)

Subject type	Message condition				
	Positive	*Negative*	*Fear*	*Control*	*All*
Willing	95	100	50	95	82·5
Unwilling	20	30	5	0	13·7
All subjects	57·5	65	27·5	47·5	

Source	*df*	*MS*	*F*
Type *A*	1	20·31	203·1*
Condition *B*	3	1·06	10·6*
$A \times B$	3	0·42	4·2*
Error	152	0·10	

*$p < 0.01$.

mind. While the traditional fear appeal was unsuccessful in increasing the signing rate (5 per cent signed), both the positive message (20 per cent) and the negative message (30 per cent) significantly increased signing behaviour. Turning to those subjects who were initially willing to be transferred to the ATU, one subject in the no-message control (5 per cent), one subject receiving the positive appeal (5 per cent) and none of the subjects receiving the negative appeal changed their minds. In marked contrast, 50 per cent of the initially willing subjects who received the traditional fear appeal did not sign up for the ATU. This 'boomerang effect' was highly significant. To summarize briefly then, the post-test behaviour of subjects in the no-message control group was consistent with their pre-test behaviour; the negative and positive appeals significantly increased signing behaviour, while the traditional fear appeal significantly reduced signing behaviour. It is worth noting that in support of the approach outlined earlier, these results correspond directly to the previously obtained changes in beliefs and attitudes.

Communicator failure

The above study demonstrates the importance of considering the theoretical relationships between message content and a given dependent variable. In addition, it shows how changes in theoretically relevant beliefs can produce changes in attitudes and behaviours. It demonstrates the importance of distinguishing between beliefs, attitudes, intentions, and behaviours, and of understanding the relationships between these variables. Finally, it points to the necessity of distinguishing between acceptance of belief statements contained in a message, *yielding* to these statements, and the *impact* effect of the statements on other beliefs that are theoretically related to the dependent variable in question.

What I have tried to argue throughout this paper is that these considerations and distinctions are essential if one is to understand the persuasive effects of a communication. Not only do these considerations allow one to develop effective communications, but they enable one to identify quickly various sources of communication failure. I personally believe that one of the main reasons for communication failure is *not* that people don't accept the information they are given, but that the information provided is inappropriate or incomplete.

For example, if a doctor wants a patient to behave in a certain way such as taking a particular prescription twice a day, he cannot assume that he can produce this behaviour by simply telling the patient that, 'I expect you to take these pills twice a day'. Assuming that this statement is accepted, it must be recalled that it represents just one of many normative beliefs about this behaviour that the patient may hold. The patient may also believe that his wife, or another doctor, or his religion thinks that he should not take the pills twice a day. Even though he may believe that 'Dr *A* thinks I should take these pills twice a day', his subjective norm might be that 'Most people who are important to me think that I should not take these pills twice a day'. Further, even if the doctor's statement does change the patient's subjective norm (ie, even if the patient does come to believe that 'most people who are important to me think I should take these pills twice a day') his intention to perform this behaviour might be completely under attitudinal control. In this case, irrespective of his subjective norm, he would only intend to engage in this behaviour if he believes that taking the pills twice a day would lead to more positive consequences and/or fewer negative consequences than not taking the pills twice a day.

To continue with this example, let us suppose that this particular behaviour is indeed under attitudinal control. In this case, the doctor could only influence the patient's behaviour by providing him with information about the advantages of taking the pills twice a day and/ or the disadvantages of not taking the pills twice a day. Notice that the information necessary to produce the desired behaviour is very specific to the behaviour being considered. Notice also that other information may have little or no influence on whether the patient takes the pills twice a day. That is, it would do relatively little good for the doctor to provide information about the pill *per se*, the nature of the patient's illness, or even the advantages of taking the pills in general. In the latter case, it should be realized that the patient may believe that taking these pills will lead to good consequences, but at the same time, he might believe that taking these pills *twice a day* will lead to negative consequences. To put this somewhat differently, when a behaviour is under attitudinal control, one must provide information that can potentially change the attitude towards the particular behaviour in question. Changing the patient's attitude towards 'Pill *X*', or even towards 'Taking Pill *X*' may have little or no influence on his attitude towards 'Taking Pill *X* twice a day'. Clearly, a person could have a positive attitude towards taking 'Pill *X* once a day' but a negative attitude towards 'Taking Pill *X* twice a day'. Once the specific behaviour and the appropriate attitude have been identified, the type of information necessary to change that attitude becomes clear. Providing any other type of information may not only have no effect on the behaviour in question, but, as in the case of the fear appeal described earlier, it may actually have an effect that is directly opposite to that intended.

To conclude, it is only recently that we have come to understand the relationships between beliefs, attitudes, intentions, and behaviours, and, as I have tried to point out throughout this paper, it is only with this knowledge that it becomes possible to understand communication effectiveness. All too often, people have pointed to the ineffectiveness of mass communication or have identified cases of communication failure when, in a sense, the communications have been entirely successful and no failure has occurred. In many of these cases, the communication did everything that it was capable of doing: people did accept the statements contained in the message.

The problem was not really one of communication failure, but one of communicator failure, ie, the failure of the communicator to link the contents of his message to the particular belief, attitude, intention, or behaviour he was trying to change. What I would like to suggest is a distinction between communication and communicator failure. If a receiver accepts the statements contained in a message, the communication process has been successful. I do not believe that we should call something a communication failure if the communicator makes erroneous assumptions about the effects of the information he presents.

Postscript

The seminar and this book are just one outcome of Charles Fletcher's Rock Carling Monograph on *Communication in Medicine* which may justly be described as a landmark in our appreciation of the importance of the subject to the practice of medicine. Fletcher divided his monograph into two parts: the first was concerned almost entirely with communication between individuals and the problems of communication which face doctors in their daily work. This looked at communication with patients, communication in hospitals, and communication between the three divisions of the NHS. The second part looked at communication with the public about medicine.

By contrast we have focused almost entirely on communication of doctors, nurses, and other health care professionals with patients. This choice was a natural one given its central importance and we have attempted to look at this aspect in greater depth. Perhaps it would be reasonable to treat the other areas in a similar fashion in the future. The choice of just one aspect is, however, indicative of the scope of the subject, albeit as Fishbein points out, many of the problems are common.

What then are the salient points that emerged on first reading of Fletcher's chapter on communication with patients? Others may identify these differently and I suppose that one's choice may in some part be influenced by one's outlook and mood. Be this as it may, the things I identified were, first and foremost, a reluctance of doctors and nurses to consider seriously that they might be failing in some large part of the consultation: the key point of clinical medicine. Secondly, little is being done to seek improvement. To quote,

> It would seem self-evident that a matter which is the chief source of dissatisfaction among our patients should have a permanent place in the teaching of medical students. I have found no reference to such teaching in the Report of the Royal Commission on Medical Education nor, with one exception, in the more

popular undergraduate textbooks on medicine. I gather from colleagues engaged on undergraduate teaching that, whereas the need for communication is usually emphasized in introductory lectures, there is little specific instruction on techniques or any continuing emphasis throughout the clinical years.

And, lastly, that the prescription of time, trouble, and empathy left me feeling dissatisfied.

This is not to imply criticism. The scope of the monograph, and of the chapter alone, mitigated against more detailed exploration. And any further exploration would have had to be multidimensional in nature and multidisciplinary in origin. For the question exposed by the points of reluctance to consider failure and the absence of teaching or guidance is—why? There are many aspects to this question which at this point I should prefer to ignore. For the purposes of this postscript, I am going to offer one answer which is that in the process of communicating with patients most of us do not know what we are doing: we know what we want to do but most of us do not know, other than intuitively, how to do it. It follows that we are unable to monitor our own performance with a view to seeking improvement. It also follows that it is not something which can be easily taught.

The five papers in this book are then a form of argument to support this point of view, and here I should like to recap some of the salient points that emerge. To the point of how bad is the situation I should like to turn to the papers by Marie Johnston and Philip Ley. Johnston in her study looked at the communication of physical and psychological feelings to nurses. As she, herself, states, she undertook a fairly severe test of communication in what, it may be added, was an extremely rigorous manner. She showed that although nurses know what patients worry about (a not surprising finding), they do not know which patients are worried or how many worries patients have. Furthermore, as has been previously shown, pain is poorly communicated along with most other physical aspects of recovery from surgery. One may question these findings but it can be argued that they are not really unexpected in that they agree with other work of a somewhat allied nature.

Ley looked first at the problem of patients' dissatisfaction with communications in hospital and using data from a number of studies showed that something between 11 and 65 per cent of patients come out of hospital feeling dissatisfied with the communications aspect of their hospital stay. The percentages vary considerably and part of this is obviously due to different samples of patients and to the different questions asked. More salutary, however, is his demonstration that the percentage of patients dissatisfied is not reduced when doctors feel that they made special efforts and indeed, when they felt that they were communicating adequately. Perhaps after all, time, trouble, and empathy are not the keys to greater success.

Coming to Peter Maguire's and Derek Rutter's paper, there is little comfort to be found in their experience with senior clinical students. Let me use Maguire's own words when he presented their paper at the seminar.

> The evidence I want to talk about is mostly derived from studies which have actually looked at what students and doctors do, rather than take their own accounts of what they do, because there are quite alarming discrepancies. Early work suggested that there were particular difficulties, not only in doctors not seeming to know always what questions to ask, but also in the behaviour they commonly used to interview. We thought that we ought to check this by taking a group of quite senior students —most of them just before finals—and giving them the task of simply finding out the nature of the patient's current problems. We deliberately chose patients who were co-operative, articulate, and likely to give an easy account of themselves. We were not, therefore, testing complex interview behaviour. We were concerned with their basic ability to get a notion of the patient's key problems.
>
> The first and most alarming thing we found was how little information the students were able to get that was either accurate or relevant. Usually they averaged around 14 items in 15 minutes, less than one item per minute, where an item would score one if it was just a symptom. So they were coming out with very little information. Why was this so? One of the major issues was the whole problem of being able to help the patient give the type of information wanted. We found that the students would let the patients ramble on matters that were not very relevant to the task. They did not seem to have been given any coherent interview procedure.
>
> The other problem that we found was that, it did not matter

whether they were organically oriented, psychologically oriented, or whatever, most of the students and doctors had an inappropriate focus. They would go for the first problem the patient volunteered. They would assume that it was the real problem, and they seemed to have no strategy which allowed them to detect that there might be other, more important problems, bothering the patient. The question style they used was usually very leading, biased, and restricting, so that the options open to the patient were very limited.

One of the very interesting things was how vague the information was that the doctors were content to accept: simple things like the exact dosage of a treatment, the dates of surgery, were left very imprecise. They seemed to have no routine way of telling the patient that they wanted precise information.

We have been talking about non-verbal behaviour. It was quite astounding the kind of gross behaviours that went, apparently, unnoticed, and unresponded to. There again, some students behaved in a manner which seriously interfered with their efforts to relate to the patient, without being in any way aware of the effect they were having.

To turn now to the subject of patient compliance with therapeutic regimes. Ley in his paper discussed compliance in medicine taking. Over-all, he showed, that in 68 studies covering patient compliance in a wide variety of instances varying from the nice to the nasty, innocuous to harmful, nearly half the patients did not follow the advice given. To extend this it is useful to consider a more recently published report by Sackett *et al.* (1975).[1] They tackled the problem of poor compliance of patients under treatment for hypertension. They undertook a randomized controlled trial to see whether compliance could be improved by either making follow-up more easy and convenient or educating patients about their disease.

Both strategies failed to yield improvement. At six months only some half of the patients were compliant and there were no significant differences between the groups. There is even a suggestion that the educational programme might have been counter-productive in one of the groups. Because of the total lack of success the study is now being extended to test a set of more behaviourally oriented strategies.

1. Sackett, D. L., Haynes, R. B., Gibson, M. D., Hackett, B., Taylor, D. W., Roberts, R. S., and Johnson, A. L. (1975). 'Randomised clinical trial of strategies for improving medication compliance in primary hypertension', *Lancet*, **i**, 1205–7.

These consist of training in home blood pressure measurement and medication charting, and the tailoring of regimes to habits and daily ritual.

At this point I feel that I have satisfactorily supported my view that most of us do not know what we are doing when we attempt to communicate. But where does this get us? I should like to think to a consideration of the other aspect of this book, which is principally concerned with what to do about it. Again I should like to recap the main themes.

Colin Fraser has provided us with a fairly detailed analysis of channels of communication and different types of communication in the face-to-face setting. In the first part of his paper he looks at overt behavioural aspects and in the second part he considers communication as meaning. Anyone reading his paper should be made more clearly aware that it is not only the words and tone that are important, but the structure of sentences, the ums and ahs, the silences, the gestures, the eye contact, play essential parts. Many might like to dismiss this as common knowledge: in reply I would offer the comment that it would be a very imperceptive or insensitive student who, after reading Fraser's analysis, continued to act in a manner such as described by Maguire: 'one student repeatedly answered "yes" to a patient in so bored a manner that the patient was reduced to silence. Another adopted an extremely casual and sprawling posture. The patient interpreted this as indifference...'

But Fraser goes further and raises questions about the relationship of the overt message and the immediate social setting and the background presuppositions which might operate. His example, 'Well, he's a typical Rotarian', is a particularly interesting one. I interpret this as something not uncommon in clinical medicine—a form of personality diagnosis arrived at intuitively and serving to describe in a word or phrase a set of characteristics, a likely manner in which a person will respond or behave, and possibly an indication of treatment or management. Fraser suggests that some of the shortcomings of communication in medical settings are due to unexamined differences in the backgrounds of doctors and patients. It is difficult to disagree with this: all that needs to be added is that from the above example we lack a suitable taxonomy!

Fraser's paper I see as the cornerstone on which to build, drawing on Maguire's and Rutter's experience and success. To me it provides much of the theory which they have applied to the medical setting, to the doctor–patient consultation. In a nutshell they set out to give the student an appropriate interviewing model, and instruct him in interviewing techniques. In this they clarify the social setting, help minimize any background presuppositions, identify different communication systems and stress attention to the message content. I think their work does much to alleviate the gloom of previous remarks and is particularly encouraging in view of Fletcher's findings concerning medical education. It can be added that other centres are developing similar educational programmes.

However, it remains to be judged whether the gloom concerning patient compliance and persuasive communication has been similarly lessened. Ley in his paper deals at length with message content. In his own words, 'If the patient does not understand what you tell him, he is not likely to follow your advice. He may be less likely to remember the advice or what was said. Part of the reason why patients were not satisfied with communications, when clinicians had tried hard to communicate with them, was because they did not understand what they were told.' While some may regard such statements as obvious, I think it is important that Ley and his colleagues have regarded them as hypotheses and proceeded to test them in a formal manner. The results are impressive but I remain somewhat uneasy about the conflict of evidence revealed by the study of Sackett and his colleagues. This conflict needs to be reconciled: possibly on the one hand we should recognize that it is not easy to generalize, on the other hand an important factor, as discussed by Fishbein, might be the patient's existing knowledge and understanding.

These remarks must not be taken in any way to diminish the contribution of Ley's paper, rather to reinforce its effect, for he shows us that a very simple model accounts for a lot of the variance in patients' dissatisfaction and in patients' non-compliances. Fishbein provides the more complex models for our thoughts of the future. In so doing he removes my unease concerning the 'old' attitude–behaviour relationship, which is patently unable to explain fairly commonplace observations. Again, he stresses the importance of message content. But possibly the most telling thing of all for everyday clinical practice is his distinction between acceptance of message content, yielding to message content, and secondary or impact effects of the message. It is appreciation of these secondary effects that, hereafter, should stop any of us thinking about a simple chain of events.

So much for this personal view, trying in part to act as observer, in part to tackle the question posed in the preamble which asked what more do we need to know in order to improve our performance as senders and receivers of messages. Five of the contributors come from disciplines other than medicine and I should like to express my thanks to them for allowing me to persuade them to contribute. I believe they have provided us with answers which, as they would admit, are not necessarily complete.

Of more importance they have provided us with a wealth of hypotheses to test. These, together with the work on medical students, should provide us with impetus and direction.

A.E.BENNETT